Everyday English for Nursing

For Baillière Tindall

Senior Commissioning Editor: Sarena Wolfaard
Project Development Manager: Dinah Thom
Project Manager: Pat Miller/Jane Dingwall
Designer: Judith Wright
Page Layout: Jim Hope (PTU Edinburgh)

Everyday English for Nursing

An English Language Resource for Nurses who are Non-native Speakers of English

Tony Grice

BPhil MA CertEd

Cartoons by Daniel Grice

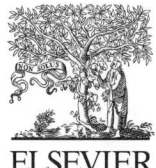

ELSEVIER

EDINBURGH LONDON NEW YORK OXFORD PHILADELPHIA ST LOUIS SYDNEY TORONTO 2003

BAILLIÈRE TINDALL
An imprint of Elsevier Limited

First published 2003
  Reprinted 2004, 2005 (twice), 2007, 2008, 2009

ISBN 978 0 7020 2687 4

British Library Cataloguing in Publication Data
A catalogue record for this book is available from the British Library

Library of Congress Cataloging in Publication Data
A catalog record for this book is available from the Library of Congress

Note
Medical knowledge is constantly changing. Standard safety precautions must be followed, but as new research and clinical experience broaden our knowledge, changes in treatment and drug therapy may become necessary or appropriate. Readers are advised to check the most current product information provided by the manufacturer of each drug to be administered to verify the recommended dose, the method and duration of administration, and contraindications. It is the responsibility of the parctitioner, relying on experience and knowledge of the patient, to determine dosages and the best treatment for each individual patient. Neither the Publisher nor the author assumes any liability for any injury and/or damage to persons or property arising from this publication.

The P ublisher

The publisher's policy is to use paper manufactured from sustainable forests

Printed in China

Contents

Please note that the topics covered in each chapter are listed below the chapter titles, and the aspects of English being tested in the accompanying exercises are given in brackets.

Foreword

There is nothing new about nurses from overseas coming to the United Kingdom to practise their profession, whether as refugees, for professional advancement, or simply for travel and the opportunity to live and work in a new environment. During the late 1930s and 1940s, nurses fleeing Nazi Germany came to the UK: in the 1950s nurses were among the new wave of those from the Caribbean, and more recently nurses from Commonwealth and British Dependent Territories countries have had the opportunity to work in the UK for short periods under the Working Holidaymaker scheme. In addition, students come to the UK to train as nurses.

These nurses were mainly competent in English and came to the UK on their own initiative. Recently, however, the rapid growth in the number of overseas nurses working in the UK is as a result of targeted recruitment, either by government-to-government agreements or by commercial recruitment agencies, from countries where English may not be the primary language. Nursing shortages, and subsequent government plans to increase the numbers of nurses working in the NHS, have meant that international nurse recruitment is one, relatively quick, way of meeting targets for growth. The independent health care sector has also experienced a nurse shortage, particularly in smaller care homes, and this sector too has turned to overseas recruitment as a solution to its problems.

The result has been a striking increase in the numbers of internationally recruited nurses in the UK. Figures from the Nursing and Midwifery Council (NMC), the professional registration body, show that in the early 1990s about one in ten new registrants were from overseas. By 2001 this had risen to four in ten, and in May 2002 NMC figures showed that overseas nurses accounted for more than half of the total of new registrants, 13 721 being admitted to the Register out of 41 656 who applied for UK registration. Significant source countries include the Philippines, South Africa, India, Australia and Zimbabwe.

These recruits are an essential part of the nursing workforce. One London NHS Trust quoted in Buchan (2003) reported employing nurses from 68 countries, and many small independent sector employers could not function effectively on UK-trained nurses alone. In short, international nurse recruitment has moved from short-term fix to planned long-term strategy.

The experiences of these new international recruits are, like those of their colleagues before them, very mixed. Some report positive experiences which have allowed them to progress in their profession in the UK, while others have been exploited by unscrupulous recruiters and employers. Some have experienced racism in the workplace and from their host communities; many others have found that they can contribute personally and professionally to our multicultural society and environment of care, and that their colleagues value this. The NHS Code of Practice (2001), the Independent Health Care Association recommendations for supervised practice programmes (2002) and the Royal College of Nursing's guide to good practice in international recruitment (2002) have done much to promote ethical recruitment practice.

But the main challenges reported by the recruits, their employers and their host colleagues are those of clinical and cultural difference, and above all, of language competency. The ability to communicate easily in English is absolutely essential if the value of international recruits is to be recognised by their host colleagues and those for whom they care – nursing is, above all, about communication, often on sensitive issues and in life-threatening situations. Hard-pressed UK nurses who are supporting and mentoring international recruits alongside their everyday responsibilities for patient care can understandably feel frustrated when communication difficulties arise, as shown by reports – some exaggerated – in professional journals and the national press, highlighting difficulties in the English language skills of some nurses.

In March 2001, the NMC's predecessor body, the United Kingdom Central Council for Nursing, Midwifery and Health Visiting, decreed that all nurses trained outside the European Union and from countries where English was not the language of nursing education must achieve a satisfactory score in the IELTS (International English Language Testing System) before being considered for admission to the UK Register. There is no power to require language competency from nurses from European Union/European Economic Area countries.

How are nurses prepared for the demands of effective communication in English? Some NHS recruiters and employers have set up their own in-house language proficiency courses, particularly those who recruit from Spain and the Philippines through a government-to-government agreement. Others use a variety of education providers and draw on the experiences of earlier international recruits to ensure that formal English teaching is supplemented by an introduction to local accent, idioms, and colloquial English, which is often ignored by conventional courses. Not all patients, and not all UK nurses, speak what we might call 'Queen's English' or have cut-glass accents reminiscent of an RAF

Officer in a British 1940s war movie, particularly when using a variety of euphemisms for intimate bodily functions. We need to address this in language programmes and in the adaptation or supervised practice programmes which may be required by the NMC before a nurse is admitted to the Register.

This book will supplement the programmes mentioned above, and will be essential for those who receive no employer support with language familiarisation. Nurses who have achieved the required IELTS standard and those from EU countries will also find it useful. It is above all a practical book – as the author says, it could be stuffed into a bag for study on the bus on the way home – particularly appropriate for those who have many other pressures of living and working in a new country. Its greatest strength is that it works through recognisable situations across the whole spectrum of nursing, and the exercises cover a range of issues from emergency care, through nursing procedures and medical conditions, to talking about death and dying. At the same time, the examples provide an insight into the working of the NHS, current nursing issues, career development, and the multicultural society that is the UK today.

Internationally recruited nurses are here to stay. They have much to offer patients and much to teach their UK colleagues, and this book responds in a fresh and lively way to their needs, and those of their colleagues, for safe, effective communication skills as the key to this.

Dee Borley
RCN Nurseline
Royal College of Nursing

References:
Buchan, J. Here to stay? International nurses in the UK (2003) London: RCN.
Nursing and Midwifery Council, May 2002.
Code of Practice for NHS employers involved in international recruitment of healthcare professionals (2002) London: Department of Health.
Supervised practice programmes for internationally recruited nurses; independent sector recommendation (2002) London: Independent Healthcare Association/Registered Nursing Homes Association.
Internationally recruited nurses: good practice guide for health care employers and RCN negotiators (2002) London: RCN.

Preface

For a long time, health services in English-speaking countries have bolstered their workforces with employees who are not native speakers of English. Sometimes, as if the jobs they do weren't difficult enough, the fact that English is not the language these employees grew up with, causes problems. In the work of healing and tending the sick, where communicating information, observations and instructions play such a vital role, misunderstandings due to language are not minor things. Healthcare professionals have been indicating a need for language support and training for some time and this book is a response to that. It aims to provide non-native speakers of English with an opportunity to practise some of the English that is written and spoken in hospitals.

Between 2000 and 2002, I visited Eastern Europe and South-East Asia where I met nurses who had just been recruited into the UK's beleaguered National Health Service (NHS). Despite the fact that these nurses had been through a selection process and their English language competence assessed and deemed adequate, they were still worried about how they would get on with the language when the time came to actually do the job. They had two fears. The first was that they would not be able to understand hospital documentation. And the second was that they would not be able to talk with real-life British people because they wouldn't be able to understand accents, dialects and idioms. This book attempts to provide these professionals with some of what they say they need – practice and exposure to the kinds of English they encounter in their work – abbreviated written English on clinical records and the spoken English of the patients they tend.

People using this book probably have little time to attend language classes and need something they can use without a teacher if need be. *Everyday English for Nursing* has been designed with self-study in mind. It is written in such a way that it questions and guides rather than teaches and instructs. Though it can be easily used as a course book or supplement to a course in a conventional language classroom, it can also be stuffed in a bag and pulled out for use during spare moments in the canteen or on the bus home.

I am happy to acknowledge the help I have received in researching and writing this book, in particular Suraya Suffian for her photographs and Daniel Grice for his cartoons and drawings. The original idea for the book came from Sevda Tsevetanova of the University of Rousse in Bulgaria, who also provided encouragement and gave me hospitality when I was in that country. I received invaluable help from Justin Shanahan and the nurses of Ward 4 at Broadgreen Hospital, Liverpool and from numerous medical and language teaching professionals who checked the material that appears in the book for authenticity and accuracy.

Bacup, Lancashire, 2003

Abbreviations

ADL   activities of daily living
AIDS   acquired immune deficiency syndrome
BMR   basal metabolic rate
BP   blood pressure
C/O   (in the) care of
CVA   cerebrovascular accident (stroke)
D/C   discontinued
DOB   date of birth
GP   general practitioner
HIV   human immunodeficiency virus
IM   intramuscular
(L)   left
LS   left side
N/A   not applicable
NWB   non-weight-bearing
OOB   out of bed
op   operation
ORS   oral rehydration salts
p.a.   per annum – every year
PMH   previous medical history
PTA   prior to admission
PTA   post traumatic amnesia
qh   every hour
ql   as much as one pleases
(R)   right
RCN   Royal College of Nursing
RS   right side
RTA   road traffic accident
TPR   temperature pulse respiration

The structure of the book and how to use it

It is assumed that people using this book have a 'higher intermediate' to 'advanced' level of fluency in English (IELTS 5.0 and above).

Because the emphasis is on practice rather than instruction, the book consists mostly of exercises. There is a little passive reading but a lot of the texts offered for reading and comprehension are simultaneously exercises for practising grammar and vocabulary so that the reader stays as actively engaged as possible.

Each chapter is in two parts. The first part contains the reading and the exercises and the second part the answers to the exercises, along with some comments on the answers that the reader might find useful. This is to make self-checking an easy and productive part of the process of learning and consolidating. Almost all the exercises can be self-checked. However, there are also exercises called 'Further Practice' which are open to individual styles of note-writing and cannot therefore be self-checked. Teachers might find 'Further Practice' exercises a useful classroom tool. Model answers are given in cases where there is more than one way of saying something.

Texts, exercises and vocabulary get harder as the book progresses. Because the language the book practises aims for authenticity, it is the medical context that dictates the language, not the other way around. Chapters in the second part of the book are organised into medical themes rather than language items, so that things like verb tenses, prepositions and articles are practised throughout the book – not in any one particular spot.

Tony Grice

Part One

The National Health Service in the UK

Chapter One

The problem

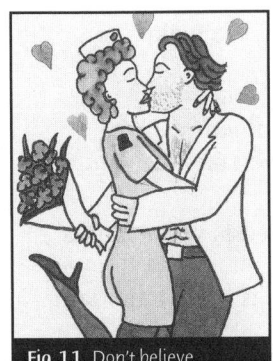

Fig. 1.1 Don't believe everything you see on TV.

Nurses in television soap operas and teenage novels are often romantic heroes and heroines. Even though they are towers of strength, they will still fall hopelessly in love with handsome doctors, weep with the pain of a broken heart when their love affair goes wrong but smile in quiet triumph when they save the life of a child who has been rushed in to A&E. You would think that everyone would want to be a nurse. But no. The truth is that though things are getting much better, the job has become unpopular and now many nurses want to get out of the profession as fast as they can. If only real life were like television!

What has gone wrong? The following letter is from a nurse who believes he knows the answer to this question.

VOCABULARY

to put upon: to exploit and ask too much.

where is the money coming from?: in the letter this question expresses an ultra-practical attitude.

an allowance: pocket money or regular income from a (rich) relative.

overdrawn: to have drawn more money from your bank account than you had in it.

to fool (themselves): to tell (themselves) something which is not true.

Dear Colleague,

I can tell you who is causing the crisis. We are! The nurses! We nurses accept the staff shortages and try to do the impossible. We allow employers <u>to put upon</u> us. We accept unpaid overtime and we accept punishment when we make understandable mistakes.

In my clinic I see 105 patients with various fractures in only 4 hours. The morning clinic finishes two-and-a-half hours after the afternoon clinic begins. I get no tea break, no meal break and it is usual practice to leave late in the afternoons.

We must stop <u>fooling</u> ourselves that being respected is what counts. A bank manager said to me, because I was <u>overdrawn</u> again, 'look – you may be a nice person who does a very important job, and society needs you, but <u>where is the money coming from</u>?'

Florence Nightingale did nurses a great disservice by only employing girls from 'good' families where Daddy paid for his daughter's training. She got <u>an allowance</u> of course and the best nurses were totally obedient and knew their place.

Yours faithfully,
PAUL JENNER

Fig. 1.2 Furiously Yours, Paul Jenner RN.

Exercise 1a   In this exercise extracts are taken from the letter you have just read. After each extract there are three sentences (a, b & c). Say which of the three sentences is closest in meaning to the extract.

1   The writer of the letter says: 'We nurses accept the staff shortages'. What does he mean?
Either: a. We don't mind the present situation.
    Or: b. We do nothing about the present situation.
    Or: c. We cannot live with the present situation.

2   'We try to do the impossible' means:
Either: a. We are asked to do amazing things.
    Or: b. Even when we know we can't do something, we still try.
    Or: c. We never succeed at what we do.

3   When the writer says 'We accept punishment when we make understandable mistakes' he means:
Either: a. We blame others when something goes wrong.
    Or: b. It's all our fault and we deserve the punishment we get.
    Or: c. It's not our fault we make mistakes, but we take the blame anyway.

4   'We must stop fooling ourselves that being respected is what counts' means:
Either: a. We are stupid to think that getting respect is more important than, say, money.
    Or: b. We must stop thinking we are respected. We aren't.
    Or: c. We are being stupid when we think we are being clever.

5   When the writer's bank manager asks 'Where is the money coming from?' he means:
Either: a. Who pays you?
    Or: b. How do you want to pay – cash, cheque or credit card?
    Or: c. You don't earn enough.

6   'Florence Nightingale did nurses a great disservice' means:
Either: a. Florence Nightingale did a lot for nurses.
    Or: b. Florence Nightingale refused to help nurses.
    Or: c. Florence Nightingale did no favours to nurses.

Exercise 1b   Practise the vocabulary that is used in the nurse's letter by filling in the spaces in the following sentences from the options a, b, c and d.

1   Nurses have to try to do .... things.
a. the impossible
b. impossible
c. this impossible
d. impossibly

2   The writer's patients have .... of fractures.
a. variety
b. various
c. a variety
d. varied

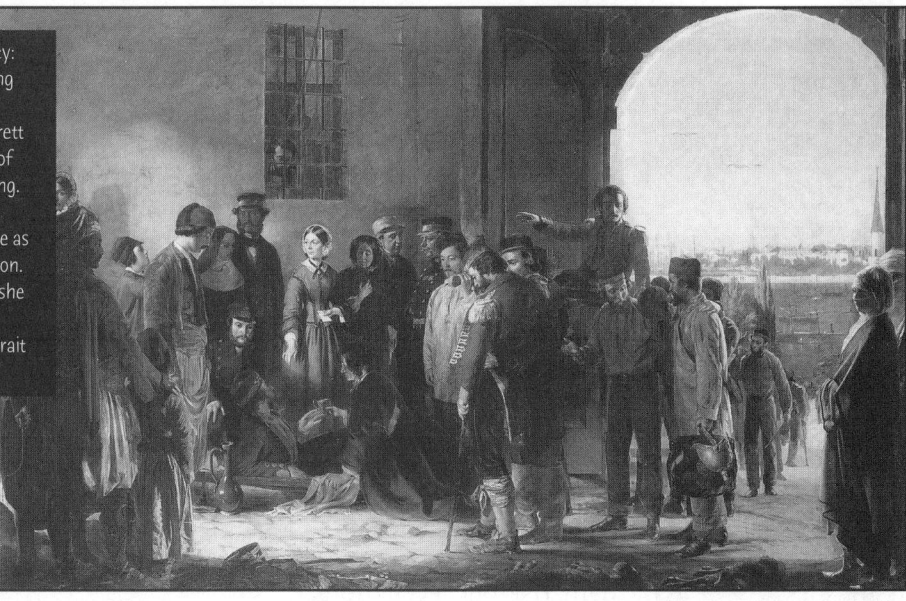

Fig. 1.3 The Mission of Mercy: Florence Nightingale receiving the wounded at Scutari. This famous painting by Jerry Barrett represents the popular view of the founder of modern nursing. However, recent biographies describe Florence Nightingale as a difficult and obsessive person. Some nurses are now saying she did nursing no favours. By courtesy of the National Portrait Gallery, London.

3 The writer thinks we have .... ourselves for too long.
a. fooled
b. fooling
c. foolish
d. fool

4 His bank won't let him .... any further.
a. overdrawn
b. overdraft
c. overdraw
d. overdrew

5 In the past, ... in nurses was a virtue.
a. obedience
b. obedient
c. obey
d. obeyed

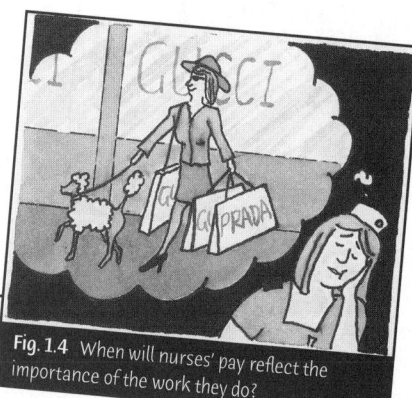

Fig. 1.4 When will nurses' pay reflect the importance of the work they do?

Exercise 1c

In the following text, choose a word from each of the brackets which fits in the space.

Many nurses in Britain say that the profession .... (are, is, were) held back by pay and status. They say that the National Health Service (NHS) is still conservative .... (mind, to mind, minded), that nurses are still subordinate ...... (by, with, to) doctors and that their professional judgement .... (do, don't, does) not get enough respect. They say that .... (though, if, when) Florence Nightingale's heart was ...... (in, on, at) the right place, she has helped to keep an .... (out dated, undated, up to date) image of the profession. They say that it is time to .... (rid, riddance, get rid) of the Florence Nightingale .... (pictorial, imagine, image) and that ...... (nurses, nurse, nurses') pay should reflect the .... (important, importantly, importance) of the work they do.

Working conditions and the crisis

at risk: in danger.

trolley: temporary bed on wheels for moving patients around.

overflowing: too many – not enough space.

to be stuck: to be unable to get out, move.

retention (from to retain): keeping nurses in the profession.

to be put off: to decide not to do something (e.g. train to be a nurse) because it is made unattractive.

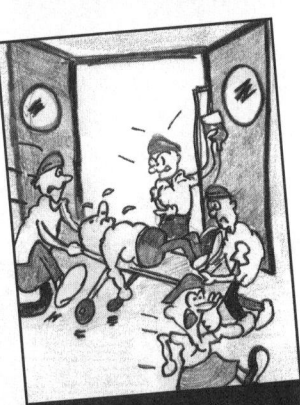

Fig. 1.5 Under pressure.

Nurses working in the NHS say that the present crisis is not just a matter of pay but also of working conditions and job satisfaction. Overcrowding in the hospitals, they say, is preventing them from doing their jobs properly and is sometimes even putting patients <u>at risk</u>.

Describing the situation at her hospital, one nurse said, 'The number of patients has been rising and, partly because of the nurse shortages, there are fewer beds. Patients become backed up in A&E and it is very, very common to see every corridor full of people waiting on <u>trolleys</u> – the department is often full to <u>overflowing</u>. Nearly 60% of the hospital's admissions arrive as emergencies – and almost always they have to wait on trolleys before a bed becomes free. Then, for those who need further hospital care, there is often a long wait before they can be moved to an in-patient ward. Last Monday, for example, 14 people were <u>stuck</u> in A&E waiting for a bed. Some had been waiting for the whole weekend.'

Because of the demand for surgical beds, hospital staff have difficult decisions to make about who to get ready for surgery, and there is a daily risk of cancellations.

Though most nurses say that poor pay and conditions have led to the recruitment and <u>retention</u> crisis in nursing, some add that modern training is too academic. They criticise recent changes in training for putting too much emphasis on academic qualifications and too little on practical skills. Many would-be nurses who do not have a strong academic interest have been <u>put off</u> and training nurses in the classroom rather than at the bedside has also led to fewer trainee nurses being available on the wards.

A report from the Government's Social Affairs Unit said, 'There is too much emphasis on status, managerial skills and the technical skills for operating medical equipment and not enough emphasis on the traditional role of nurses – comforting, feeding and bathing the sick.'

Exercise 1d

Check your understanding of the text above by answering these questions:

1 We are told 'there are fewer beds in hospitals' (2nd paragraph). This is because:
a. there are more patients now.
b. of more than one reason.
c. there are too few nurses.

2 'Patients' who 'become backed up' (2nd paragraph) are people:
a. with back injuries.
b. who have changed their minds about staying in hospital.
c. waiting their turn.

3 There are people who 'had been waiting for the whole weekend' (2nd paragraph). These are:
a. patients who had been waiting since Saturday morning.

b. patients who waited over Sunday.

d. patients who were waiting until Saturday morning.

4 Hospital staff have to decide 'who to get ready for surgery' (3rd paragraph). In other words they:

a. have to decide which of the staff are going to work in surgery.

b. can't decide who goes first.

c. have to work out which patients have priority.

5 'Would be nurses' (4th paragraph) are:

a. people training to be nurses.

b. people who might become nurses.

c. people who used to be nurses.

Agency nurses: a sticking plaster solution

VOCABULARY

a sticking plaster solution: a temporary solution.

morale: spirit and sense of well-being.

stressed: unhappy and overworked.

flexibly: quickly adapting to changes.

cover: someone who does your work when you are not able to.

competent: able, capable.

incentives: encouragement, reward.

continuity: unbroken line.

The situation in the hospitals has led to a <u>stressed</u> workforce that suffers poor <u>morale</u> and to a profession that is not attractive to potential new recruits. The gaps in staffing are filled by the extensive use of private agency staff. This is expensive, sometimes very expensive. One hospital manager in the north of England said 'the situation has become so bad that some NHS Trusts in Leeds are paying private agency nurses to travel from London (about 200 miles) because they are unable to recruit nurses from the local area.'

He said, 'In the past, hospitals used agency nurses to top up nursing levels, but now we have no alternative but to rely on them day to day to make sure we are adequately staffed. We are very short of money but we're having to pay private nurses very high rates of pay just to keep wards open.'

'To attract nurses back into the NHS they must be paid properly and be able to combine work with family responsibilities. We're doing things like trying to get people who are out of nursing practice back in, getting out to supermarkets and holding road shows, offering term-time contracts, job shares, and generally work more <u>flexibly</u> than in the past. But this all takes time and our problems are now.'

In the meantime, the hospitals have to find nurse <u>cover</u>. Often, that comes from temporary nurses. They are of two kinds – bank nurses, who are a pool of NHS nurses, and nurses from commercial agencies. Hospitals tend to have their own 'bank', made up of nurses who work at the hospital and who want to do extra shifts or simply work part-time as and when shifts come up. The fear has been raised that temporary nurses are working in areas with which they are unfamiliar, and placing patients at risk.

One ward sister said: 'We have had people turn up for duty when, in the opinion of the ward sister, they have not been <u>competent</u> in that area. So they have been sent back to the agency.' She also said that at her hospital they have had to increase pay rates for specialist areas such as cardiology and intensive care, because agencies are offering huge <u>incentives</u> to staff to go to London and work for them there.

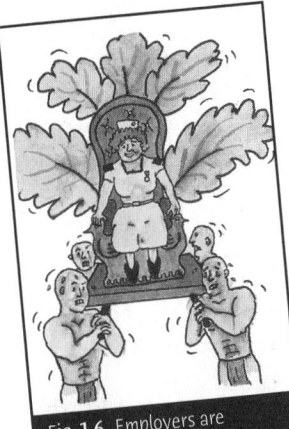

Fig. 1.6 Employers are offering all sorts of incentives.

In an interview with the BBC, Liz Jenkins, Assistant General Secretary of the Royal College of Nursing (RCN) pointed out that 'in addition to the fact that employing an agency nurse costs more than employing a staff nurse, when you get too many agency nurses, you get no <u>continuity</u> of care. The patient in their bed sees a different person every day who doesn't understand their condition, who may not even know much about the hospital they work in.'

Exercise 1e

Using words which are in the vocabulary lists in front of the previous two areas of text, complete the following sentences. The words will have to be changed in some small way (the first one is done as an example).

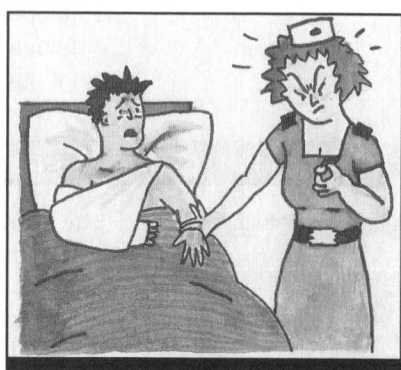

Fig. 1.7 People do not work happily on low pay.

a. The ward began to fill up and by eight o'clock the queue had .... into the corridor. (meaning: what happens when there is no space).
   Answer: The ward began to fill up and by eight o'clock the queue had <u>overflowed</u> into the corridor.

b. She had no idea about how to do the job and was sacked for being .... (meaning: not able to work effectively).

c. Low pay is never a good ...... to work hard. (meaning: a reward which encourages or motivates you).

d. She has worked in this post for a .... period of four years. (meaning: unbroken).

e. Because of the many problems in the NHS, ... nurses is very difficult. (meaning: keeping staff).

Exercise 1f

Here is a summary of what you have just read. The articles (a, an, the, some) have been left out. Complete the summary, putting a word into each space (if necessary):

...... nurses are finding it difficult working in .... NHS hospitals .... wards are overcrowded and understaffed. There is .... problem with recruitment and training and, in order to adequately staff .... wards, many hospitals have to use .... agency nurses, which means not only do they have to pay more, but .... standard of patient care is lowered.

Pay: the facts

In April 2002, nurses' salaries in the UK were increased. Compared with nurses in some other countries, nurses in the UK may seem well paid. However, to get a fair picture you need to compare the figures with the UK cost of living.

Read the following information about the rates of pay and, with that information, complete the table that follows it. Amounts of money are written in words; when you complete the table, use numbers.

Exercise 1g

Nurses' salaries are on scales in nine grades. The salaries rise in the grades according to experience and length of service. Salaries also vary depending on qualifications and medical specialism.

Unqualified auxiliary nurses are on three grades. The bottom of the scale in Grade A is nine thousand seven hundred and thirty-five pounds per annum (p.a.) and the top of the scale of the highest unqualified grade is sixteen thousand and five pounds p.a. The top salary on Grade B is thirteen thousand four hundred and eighty-five pounds.

When fully qualified staff nurses on Grade D reach the top of the scale they can expect to get seventeen thousand six hundred and seventy pounds. If they move up a grade to E the maximum pay increases to twenty thousand six hundred and fifty-five pounds.

The bottom of the Junior Sister pay scale (Grade F) is eighteen thousand nine hundred and seventy pounds, which is less than the highest paid Senior Staff nurses who earn twenty thousand six hundred and fifty-five pounds.

Grade G rises from twenty two thousand three hundred and eighty-five pounds to twenty six thousand three hundred and forty pounds. The top salaries of specialist nurses on Grade H are twenty nine thousand nine hundred and ninety pounds. Senior nurses can earn thirty-one thousand eight hundred and thirty pounds p.a. and the least they will earn is twenty-seven thousand six hundred and ninety-five pounds.

Unqualified nurse
Grade A
...... – £12 220

Unqualified nurse
Grade B
£11 455 – ......

Unqualified nurse
Grade C
£13 040 – ......

Staff Nurse
Grade D
£16 005 – ......

Senior Staff Nurse
Grade E
£17 105 – ......

Junior Sister
Grade F
...... – £24 565

Ward Manager
Grade G
£22 385 – ......

Nurse with specialist role
Grade H
£25 005 – ......

Senior Nurse
Grade I
...... – ......

Exercise 1h

Which of the following statements are true?

a. A nurse's salary increases the more experience the nurse has.
b. A nurse's salary decreases the higher up the grade the nurse is.
c. A nurse's salary is on three grades.
d. A nurse on Grade D is at the top of the scale.
e. Nurses on Grade D are paid £16 005.

f. A nurse on grade D gets no more than £17670.
g. The lowest paid Junior Sisters receive as much as the highest paid Senior Staff Nurses.
h. The lowest paid Junior Sisters get more than the highest paid Senior Staff Nurses.
i. Grade A nurses are at the bottom of the scale.
j. Grade A nurses are at the foot of the table.
k. Grade A nurses are paid on two scales.

Answers and comments on the language

Exercise 1a

1 The best choice is **b**. The writer is angry that nurses don't do anything about their working conditions. Option **a** is not the best choice because you can accept a bad situation but still 'mind' it. To 'live with' a bad situation (option **c**) is to accept it without liking it.

2 The best choice is **b**. Although nurses are asked to do 'impossible' things, these are not 'amazing' things (option **a**) which are more likely to be things like miracles, magic tricks or walking on water. It is possible to succeed at doing 'impossible' things when the word is used in this exaggerated way (option **c**).

3 The best choice is **c**. The writer means that the mistakes we make are understandable because anyone who is asked to do impossible things would make the same mistakes, so he is saying it is not the nurses' fault.

4 The best choice is **a**. Something that 'counts' is something that is important. To 'fool yourself' is to persuade yourself that something is true when it is not.

5 The best choice is **c**. When the bank manager asks 'where is the money coming from?' he is exclaiming that the writer (of the letter) simply does not have enough money.

6 The best choice is **c**. A 'disservice' is the opposite of a favour (or a service) and doing 'no favours' for somebody often means doing a disservice rather than doing nothing.

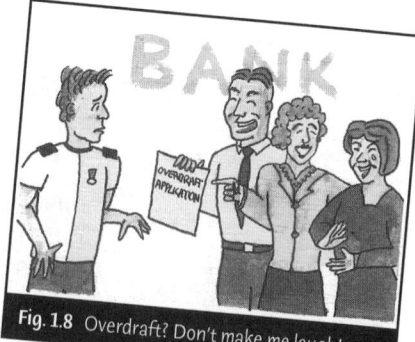

Fig. 1.8 Overdraft? Don't make me laugh!

Exercise 1b

1 b. Nurses have to try to do <u>impossible</u> things.

2 c. The writer's patients have <u>a variety</u> of fractures.

3 a. The writer thinks we have <u>fooled</u> ourselves for too long.

4 c. His bank won't let him <u>overdraw</u> any further.

5 a. In the past, <u>obedience</u> in nurses was a virtue.

Exercise 1c

Many nurses in the UK say that the profession <u>is</u> held back by pay and status. They say that the NHS is still conservative <u>minded</u>, that they are still subordinate <u>to</u> doctors and that their professional judgement <u>does</u> not get enough respect.

They say that, <u>though</u> Florence Nightingale's heart was <u>in</u> the right place, she has helped to keep an <u>outdated</u> image of the profession. They say that it is time to <u>get rid</u> of the Florence Nightingale <u>image</u> and that <u>nurses'</u> pay should reflect the <u>importance</u> of the work they do.

Exercise 1d

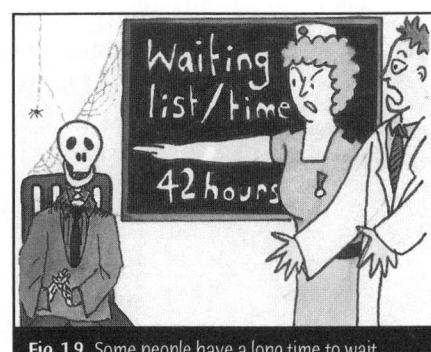

Fig. 1.9 Some people have a long time to wait.

1 b. The text tells us that there are fewer beds <u>partly</u> because of the nurse shortage – which means that this is only one reason but that there are others.

2 c. To 'back up' has a number of different uses in English. For example, it can mean 'to reverse'. 'To back out' can mean to 'change your mind' as in option **b**.

3 a. When does a weekend start? Friday night? Saturday morning? The prepositions 'since', 'over' and 'until' are important here. Option **b** is true but not the best choice.

4 c. The important thing is who is 'who' in the sentence – staff or patients? Option **a** might be right if the sentence read: 'Hospital staff have to decide who gets ready for surgery'. Option **b** doesn't tell us that some patients will not get to surgery – it only considers the order they will be in. Option **c** means to decide who is most important from a surgical point of view.

5 b. Normally, a person who is a 'would-be' something wants to become something. The story called 'The Man Who Would Be King' is about a man who wants to be a king. In the text, 'would-be nurses' are people who are thinking about becoming nurses.

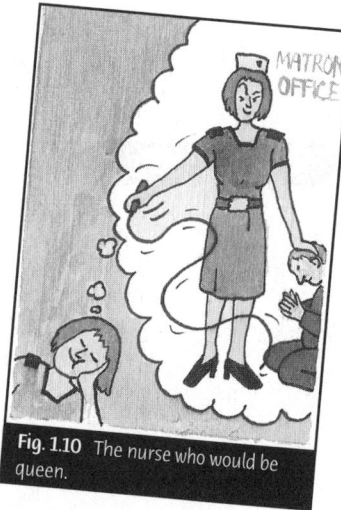

Fig. 1.10 The nurse who would be queen.

Exercise 1e

b. She had no idea about how to do the job and was sacked for being <u>incompetent</u>. Note that you make 'competent' into a negative by adding the prefix 'in-'.

c. Low pay is never a good <u>incentive</u> to work hard.

d. She has worked in this post for a <u>continuous</u> period of four years.

e. Because of the many problems in the NHS, <u>retaining</u> nurses is very difficult.

Exercise 1f

Some (or no article) nurses are finding it difficult working in no article NHS hospitals. The (or no article) wards are overcrowded and understaffed. There is a problem with recruitment and training and, in order to adequately staff the (or no article) wards, many hospitals have to use no article agency nurses, which means that not only do they have to pay more, but the standard of patient care is lowered.

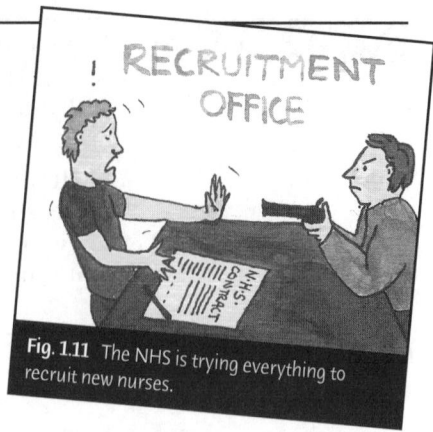

Fig. 1.11 The NHS is trying everything to recruit new nurses.

Exercise 1g

Unqualified nurse
Grade A
£9735–£12 220

Unqualified nurse
Grade B
£11 455–£13 485

Nurse
Grade C
£13 040–£16 005

Staff Nurse
Grade D
£16 005–£17 670

Senior Staff Nurse
Grade E
£17 105–£20 655

Junior Sister
Grade F
£18 970–£24 565

Ward Manager
Grade G
£22 385–£26 340

Nurse with specialist role
Grade H
£25 005–£29 990

Senior Nurse
Grade I
£27 695–£31 830

Exercise 1h

a. is true. Note the structure of the sentence – X happens the more Y happens. For example: 'the risk of cancer increases the more someone smokes.'
b. is not true.
c. is not true. There are nine grades.
d. is not true. There is a scale in each grade so it is possible for a nurse on Grade D to be at the top of the scale in Grade D but not automatically. Most nurses aren't.
e. is not true. Some nurses (not all) on Grade D are paid £16 005.
f. is true. £17 670 is the top of the scale.
g. is not true.
h. is not true.
i. is not true. They are at the bottom of the table.
j. is true. The 'bottom' of the table and the 'foot' of the table are the same place.
k. is not true. Note the differences between 'scale', 'grade' and 'table'. Here, the 'table' is divided into 'grades' and there is a 'scale' in each 'grade'.

Chapter Two

Foreign nurses and the NHS

UK hospitals need foreign nurses

At the beginning of 2002, there were between 8000 and 17 000 nursing vacancies in NHS hospitals. Because it is not possible to fill these vacancies with UK nationals, the NHS has to recruit nurses from abroad.

At present, foreign nurses and midwives from at least 24 different countries are registered in the UK. Amongst other places they come from Finland, Ireland, Germany, Spain, eastern Europe, South Africa, Australia, Malaysia, the Philippines, Singapore and New Zealand.

Between 35 000 and 40 000 foreign nurses are currently working in the UK, which is 10% of the total number of nurses employed by the NHS. The NHS receives 1000 new enquiries every week. At the moment, only 35% of foreign applicants are accepted at their first attempt. Nurses from countries outside the European Union (EU) have to take an adaptation course before they can be registered. Many applicants are rejected until they improve their English language skills.

Nurses are leaving countries where they are also badly needed and some countries are asking the UK not to take any more of their nurses. NHS Trusts have agreed only to recruit from countries where there is a clear nursing surplus.

A spokeswoman for the NMC said, 'we are currently looking at ways we can fast-track some applicants without compromising existing standards.'

Fig. 2.1 Fast tracking.

Exercise 2a

From your reading of 'UK hospitals need foreign nurses' answer the following questions. In each question the choices of a, b and c are all correct, but one is better than the others. Choose which best expresses the meaning of the text:

1 First paragraph. How many nursing vacancies are there?
a. As many as 17 000.
b. As few as 17 000.
c. Not more than 17 000.

2 Second paragraph. The overseas nurses and midwives:
a. come from various countries.
b. come from more than one country.
c. come from all over the world.

3 Third paragraph.
a. Some applicants are turned down.
b. Some applicants are not accepted.
c. A lot of applications are refused.

4 Third paragraph.
a. English language skills are rather important for the job.
b. English language skills are useful for the job.
c. English language skills are essential for the job.

5 Fourth paragraph.
a. NHS Trusts don't want nurses from countries where they are already badly needed.
b. NHS Trusts have refused to accept nurses from countries where they are badly needed.
c. NHS Trusts have responded to requests from some countries not to recruit from them.

Exercise 2b

The following words appear in the text. Adapt them to fit the spaces in the sentences:
vacancy, compromise, fast-track, suffer, reject, surplus

a. It is important not .... standards.
b. The need is urgent so some candidates can be ....
c. The NHS has been .... staff shortages for a long time.
d. It will be a long time before .... are all filled.
e. A .... applicant can still apply the following year.
f. It is only fair to recruit from countries with a .... of nurses.

Job advertisements

UK employers do not usually take direct applications from overseas nurses. Normally this is done through an agency in the countries from which nurses are being recruited. Here are some examples of jobs currently being advertised through an agency:

Nursing Opportunities in the UK

Quality Recruitment Ltd is offering a variety of positions in all areas of the UK. We have the following posts available now. (Please note: applicants should be _eligible_ to register with UKCC.)

For an application form, please send a brief copy of your CV to: Quality Recruitment Ltd, 3 Arnold Lane, Islingborough, London WC1.

1. General Medicine

Research, tradition and excellent pathways for promotion in large teaching hospital in the heart of London. Great subsidised accommodation.

2. Rehabilitation Staff

Highly regarded hospital on London outskirts seeks experienced rehabilitation staff for their Rehab. Unit. Friendly, open staff plus good working conditions. Attractive benefits such as season ticket loans, pension schemes, restaurant, sporting facilities and crèche available.

3. Clinical Nurse Specialist – Urology

Small friendly Central London hospital. Post-basic course in Urology required. Position requires a self-starter and autonomous practitioner as will run own clinic and department.

4. Accident and Emergency

Large hospital in outlying London area seeks nurses for both senior and junior positions in Accident and Emergency. Flexible working, holiday pay and preferential rates at local gym.

VOCABULARY

eligible: qualifications and experience are the right ones.

Advertisement 1
pathways for promotion: different ways to go forward in a career.
heart of London: somewhere in the middle of the city.
subsidised accommodation: part of the rent is paid by the employer.

Advertisement 2
highly regarded: with a good reputation.
London outskirts: the residential outer parts of London.
benefits: advantages.
season ticket loans: we will lend you the money to buy train/bus tickets for periods of time – one month, a year, etc.
crèche: nursery/kindergarten.

Advertisement 3
post-basic course: a course which is a step above the basic course.
self-starter: someone who is motivated and doesn't need to be told what to do.
autonomous: independent, working alone.

Advertisement 4
to seek: to look for.
flexible working: hours that are not regular.
preferential rates: cheaper than other people have to pay.

Exercise 2c

Fill in the spaces in the text below with words from the vocabulary lists:

Many of the .... (meaning: jobs available) offer rapid promotion and opportunities for personal development. To attract the right .... (meaning: people who apply), employers are offering all kinds of .... (meaning: advantages/extras) including pensions, accommodation at .... (meaning: cheaper than other people have to pay), subsidised travel to and from work and home, ... (meaning: nursery for young children) facilities and so on.

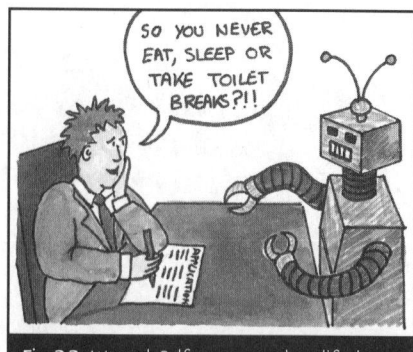

Fig. 2.2 Wanted: Self-starters and qualified applicants who can work autonomously.

Mostly, employers are .... (meaning: looking for) qualified and experienced nurses who can work .... (meaning: by themselves without supervision) and handle responsibilities.

There are jobs all over the country and those in London are both in the city as well as in the .... (meaning: on the edge) where the cost of living is lower.

Exercise 2d

Which of the following statements about the advertisements are true?

Advertisement 1: General Medicine
a. We provide luxury apartments for staff.
b. Cheap accommodation is provided.
c. You find your own accommodation and the employer pays for it.

Advertisement 2: Rehabilitation staff
d. The hospital is famous.
e. The job offers free transportation.
f. The job is not suitable for nurses with young children.

Advertisement 3: Clinical Nurse Specialist – Urology
g. The job involves training in urology.
h. The job demands training in urology.
i. The job involves management.

Advertisement 4: Accident and Emergency
j. There is a gym at the hospital.
k. The hospital needs nurses with only a little experience.
l. A junior nurse can apply for senior positions at this hospital.

Exercise 2e

Here are details about employment in the UK. Fill in the spaces in the text using either: by, with, on, for, to, in, from, of, then (some of these words can be used more than once).

UK employers do not usually take direct applications .... overseas nurses. If you are not currently .... the UK you need .... find a nursing agency .... your own country that has a contract .... recruit .... behalf .... a UK employer.

.... all countries you should look .... advertisements .... nursing journals and newspapers which have been placed .... agencies. If there is no agency recruiting .... it means that no UK employers are currently looking .... staff in your country. You will not need .... apply .... a work permit – UK employers will do that .... you – but you will need to register .... the UKCC.

Rossitza Bontcheva – Bulgarian nurse

VOCABULARY

to pop (something) into: 'light' colloquial expression meaning to put in.

to score: to get, gain (a mark/grade). Also: 'score a goal/points.'

to be pregnant: to be expecting a baby. Note: a woman gets/becomes pregnant.

to extend: to improve and increase.

to take up a post: to start working as.

money is tight: there is not much money.

to settle: to get organised and familiar with a new place.

This is the biography of a nurse from Bulgaria who applies for a job in the UK. Using the information in the biography, answer the questions that follow.

When she was a child, Rossitza wanted to be a doctor, not a nurse. Born on 1st July 1973 in Plovdiv, her first memories are of playing 'doctors' – her favourite game. First she used her dolls as patients and later she used her friends. While her father was lounging in front of the TV set, Rossitza would bandage his arms and legs and pop a thermometer into his mouth.

After primary school, there followed four years at 27 Secondary School I, Vazov. Rossitza worked hard but she didn't like academic work and so did not do well enough to become a doctor. However, she scored an average of 5 in the Diploma of Completed Secondary Education and this was enough for her to get into the Medical University in Sofia in 1992 to take a BSc degree in Nursing.

While she was studying, she fell in love with a medical student called Ilya Bontchev. They had a short romance and married in 1994. In some ways it was a mistake. A year later, Ilya left to work in Syria, fell in love with someone else while he was there and on 15th May 1996 Ilya and Rossitza were divorced. Rossitza was pregnant when Ilya left for Africa and on January 14th 1995 she had a son, Ivan. Rossitza kept her married name.

Rossitza's first job was at the Pirogov Emergency Hospital in Sofia. She stayed for two years, getting as much experience as possible and also extending her qualifications with a Certificate in Orthopaedic Nursing. She also studied English in her spare time and in October 1997 she passed the Cambridge FCE. She left the Pirogov in November 1997 and took up a post as staff nurse at the Alexandrovska Hospital. She also moved into a new flat at number 5, Gurov Street, Sofia 1602.

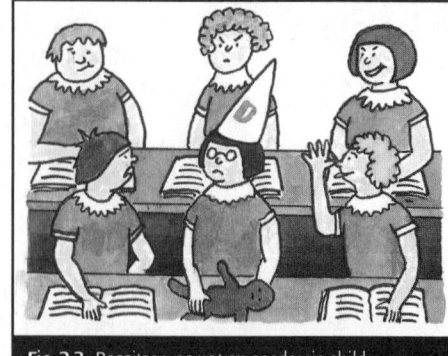

Fig. 2.3 Rossitza was not an academic child.

All this time, Ivan was growing up. It was difficult for Rossitza to be a mother and have a career. Money was tight and, when she heard that UK NHS Trusts were recruiting nurses from outside the UK, she decided to apply for a job.

Her sister was already in England and, besides, Rossitza wanted to leave behind unhappy memories and make a fresh start. She decided that if she got a job there she would go alone, settle and send for Ivan later.

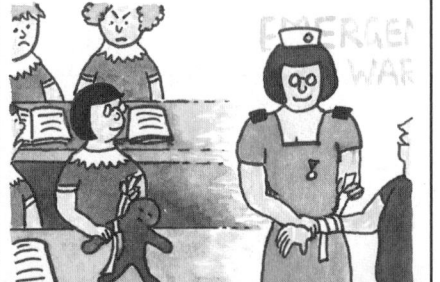

Fig. 2.4 Rossitza Bontcheva. From Plovdiv to the UK National Health Service.

Exercise 2f   **Complete each of the following sentences by choosing a, b or c.**

1   Rossitza:
   a. had a sick father.
   b. pretended her father was sick.
   c. tended her father when he was sick.

2   When Rossitza was younger she:
   a. did not want a nurse.
   b. did not want nursing.
   c. did not want to be a nurse.

3   At school, Rossitza was:
   a. an outstanding student.
   b. a willing student.
   c. a success.

4   Ilya went to Syria in:
   a. 1993.
   b. 1994.
   c. 1995.

5 Ivan was born:
a. after Rossitza's divorce.
b. before Rossitza's divorce.
c. before Rossitza was married.

6 At the Pirogov, Rossitza:
a. became better qualified.
b. became qualified.
c. qualified as a nurse.

7 Rossitza's second job was:
a. a sideways move.
b. the same as her first job.
c. higher up the ladder.

8 Money was:
a. hard to come by.
b. plentiful.
c. adequate.

This is Rossitza's CV:

Curriculum Vitae

Name:	Rossitza Bontcheva
Nationality:	Bulgarian
DOB:	1.7.73
Address:	5 Gurov Street, Sofia 1602, Bulgaria
Email:	RossB@yagoo.blg.com
Marital status:	divorced, one dependant – son (DOB: 1.14.95)

Professional qualifications:

Postgraduate Cert. in Orthopaedic Nursing (1996)
BSc Nursing at Medical University, Sofia, Bulgaria
1992–1995

English language competence:

Cambridge FCE 1997

Professional experience:

1997–present: Staff nurse (orthopaedics) at Alexandrovska Hospital, Sofia, Bulgaria. This position involves clinical management and supervision of student nurses. Also extensive use of advanced medical technology.

1995–1997: Registered nurse at Pirogov Emergency Hospital. In the second year of my employment, I specialised in orthopaedic nursing.

Exercise 2g

Which of the following statements are true?

a. Rossitza is a graduate.
b. Her degree is her most recent nursing qualification.
c. She has had fewer than two nursing jobs.
d. She has had managerial experience.
e. Rossitza is no longer a staff nurse.
f. She now works at the Pirogov Emergency Hospital.
g. She has qualifications but no experience of orthopaedic nursing.

Read this short simulated report on the problems of using nurses in hospitals who are not native speakers of English.

REPORT

Date: August 2003

PROBLEMS WITH OVERSEAS NURSES IN THE NHS

The current situation

The Nursing and Midwifery Council (NMC) says that the number of overseas nurses applying to join the UK register is rising. The NMC is worried that many of the applicants cannot speak English well enough to communicate with patients and staff. The NMC has advised the NHS that 'they need to consider carefully the level of language competence and communication skill necessary to do the job safely and effectively.'

Because good communication is an essential part of a nurse's work, overseas nurses must be competent in the following areas:

- Communicating with staff (Clear and accurate speaking and listening and understanding and recording information of a variety of different types).
- Communicating with patients (Understanding colloquial expressions, accents and dialects and being able to speak English in a clear and confident way).

Problems

There is a need to ensure protection of patients and at the same time be fair to the applicants from overseas.

Applicants from overseas should know what they are going to face in the UK.

There is a need for a consistency of standards.

There is a need to ensure that overseas nurses can adapt to the professional practices in the UK. They need to work to the same level as UK-trained practitioners.

The issues of language are the same for nurses from the Philippines as they are for nurses from France but it is difficult for the NMC to demand language competence from nurses trained in EU countries when that would contravene European laws of freedom of movement.

Recommendations

- That all non-native speaking applicants pass a language test regardless of their nationality.
- That all recruited nurses have easy access to training schemes and other professional support.

Exercise 2h

1   The report says that 'the NMC has advised the NHS'. What does this mean? (choose from a, b & c)
a. The NHS has been advised by the **NMC**.
b. The **NMC** has received advice from the NHS.
c. The NHS are advised by the **NMC**.

2   The report says that 'communication is an essential part of a nurse's work.' In other words: (choose from a, b & c)
a. all nurses communicate.
b. a nurse must communicate.
c. a nurse's work is communication.

3   One of the problems is 'a need for a consistency of standards'. This means: (choose from a, b & c)
a. standards should be the same.
b. standards could be the same.
c. standards are the same.

4   The report says that the NHS 'need to ensure that overseas nurses work to the same level as UK practitioners'. This comment is referring to: (choose from a, b & c)
a. language.
b. practices.
c. standards.

5   The 'easy access to training schemes' recommended by the report is the same as: (choose from a, b & c)
a. courses that are easy to get to.
b. courses that are easy to pass.
c. courses that can be done easily.

6   To 'contravene European laws of freedom of movement' would be to: (choose from a, b & c)
a. freely break laws set by the European movement.
b. freely move away from European laws.
c. break laws about the free movement of Europeans.

Exercise 2i

This is a list of some of the words used in the report. Put the words into the appropriate spaces in the following sentences. Each word will need to be altered in some way.

colloquial
contravene
access
applicants
competence
effective
consistency

a. Standards of work are .... by poor communication.
b. A nurse needs to be a .... communicator.
c. A nurse needs an understanding of dialects, accents, idioms and ....
d. Standards need to be ....
e. To demand language competence would be a .... of European laws.
f. The number of people .... for jobs in the NHS is rising.
g. Training schemes need to be .... to all newly recruited nurses.

Answers and comments on the language

Exercise 2a

1   The best choice is **a**. This option emphasises the fact that there are a lot of vacancies. Expressions like 'as many as' are used to emphasise how big the number is, whereas expressions like 'as few as' (option **b**) and 'not more than' (option **c**) emphasise how small the number is.

2   The best choice is **c**. The long list of countries in the article is a way to draw to the reader's attention just how many different countries the nurses come from.

3   The best choice is **c**. In the text are the words 'only 35% are accepted'. This emphasises how few applicants are accepted and therefore how many are rejected.

4   The best choice is **c**. There is a connection in the text between English language skills and being accepted for the job and option **c** expresses the importance of this connection, whereas the other two options suggest that English is not of such great importance.

5   The best choice is **c**. Options **a** and **b** are too strong. The text says that there is agreement between NHS Trusts and other countries and option **c** expresses this idea.

Exercise 2b

a. It is important not <u>to compromise</u> standards.
b. The need is urgent so some applicants can be <u>fast-tracked</u>.
c. The NHS has been <u>suffering</u> staff shortages for a long time.
d. It will be a long time before <u>vacancies</u> are all filled.
e. A <u>rejected</u> applicant can still apply the following year.
f. It is only fair to recruit from countries with <u>a surplus</u> of nurses.

Exercise 2c

Many of the <u>vacancies</u> offer rapid promotion and opportunities for personal development. To attract the right <u>applicants</u>, employers are offering all kinds of <u>benefits</u> including pensions, accommodation at <u>preferential rates</u>, subsidised travel to and from work and home, <u>crèche</u> facilities and so on.

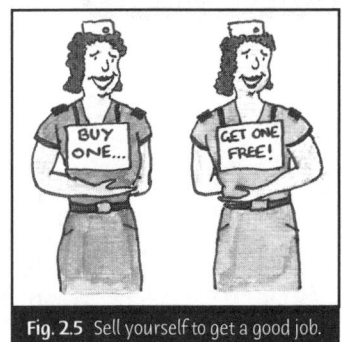

Fig. 2.5 Sell yourself to get a good job.

Mostly, employers are <u>seeking</u> qualified and experienced nurses who can work <u>autonomously</u> and handle responsibilities.

There are jobs all over the country and those in London are both in the city as well as in the <u>outskirts</u> where the cost of living is lower.

Exercise 2d

Advertisement 1: General Medicine

a. is not true. 'Great accommodation' is good accommodation, not necessarily of a luxury standard.

b. is true.

c. is not true. The employer provides the accommodation and it is 'subsidised', which means that though it is not free, it is cheap.

Advertisement 2: Rehabilitation Staff

d. is not true. 'Highly regarded' means 'well thought of' or 'respected' but not automatically 'famous'.

e. is not true. You borrow the money for season tickets from the employer.

f. is not true. A crèche is available for young children.

Advertisement 3: Clinical Nurse Specialist – Urology

g. is not true.

h. is true. Note the difference between 'involves' and 'demands'. 'The job *involves* training in urology' means that when you are employed you will get training in urology whereas 'The job *demands* training in urology' means that applicants for the job should be trained in urology.

i. is true. '…as will run own clinic' is the shortened version of: 'as the nurse will run her own clinic'. 'To run' here is 'to administer' or 'to manage'.

Advertisement 4: Accident and Emergency

j. is not true. The gym is nearby not 'at' the hospital. 'Local' means 'in the neighbourhood'.

k. is true. 'junior' means 'new to the job'.

l. is not true. The positions available for junior nurses and senior nurses are not the same ones.

Exercise 2e

UK employers do not usually take direct applications <u>from</u> overseas nurses. If you are not currently <u>in</u> the UK you need <u>to</u> find a nursing agency <u>in</u> your own country that has a contract <u>to</u> recruit <u>on</u> behalf <u>of</u> a UK employer.

<u>In</u> all countries you should look <u>for</u> advertisements <u>in</u> nursing journals and newspapers which have been placed <u>by</u> agencies. If there is no agency recruiting <u>then</u> it means that no UK employers are currently looking <u>for</u> staff in your country. You will not need <u>to</u> apply <u>for</u> a work permit – UK employers will do that <u>for</u> you – but you will need to register <u>with</u> the UKCC.

Exercise 2f

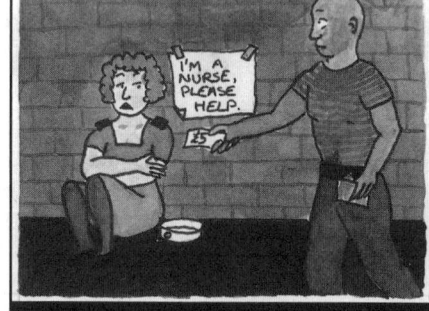

Fig. 2.6 Money is always tight.

1   **b.** Note the difference between 'pretend' and 'tend'. Rossitza played with her father and *pretended* he was sick so she could *tend* to him.

2   **c.**

3   **b.** We read that Rossitza worked hard at school but was not very successful. 'Outstanding' (option **a**) means excellent. 'Willing' (option **b**) means something like 'tries hard'.

4   **c.** Ilya went to Syria a year after their marriage in 1994.

5   **b.** Rossitza and Ilya were divorced in 1996. Ivan was born in 1995.

6   **a.** Note how a hospital can be referred to as simply 'the Pirogov' or 'the General' or 'the Queen Anne', etc. At the Pirogov Rossitza 'extended' her qualifications.

7   **c.** A 'sideways move' (option **a**) is a different job but at the same rank.

8   **a.** Note that there are a lot of different ways of saying 'I don't have much/any money' including: 'I am skint', 'I am brassick', 'I am broke', 'I am hard up', 'I am short', 'I am penniless', etc.

Exercise 2g

a. is true. Someone with a degree is 'a graduate'. Generally in UK English you graduate only from universities and colleges – not from schools. Someone who finishes school is a 'school-leaver'.

b. is not true. Note the convention of writing on CVs your most recent qualifications and jobs first and working back in time. Therefore Rossitza's most recent nursing qualification is a 'Postgraduate certificate in Orthopaedic Nursing'.

c. is not true. 'Fewer than...' means 'a smaller number than...' which would mean she has had only one job.

d. is true. She has experience of supervising other nurses.

e. is not true. The words '...to (the) present (time)' on the CV mean up to and including now.

f. is not true. She is still working at the Alexandrovska Hospital.

g. is not true. Her CV suggests that she has been employed as an orthopaedic nurse at the Pirogov.

Exercise 2h

1 a. Option **b** is the wrong way around. Option **c** gives the impression that the NHS regularly advises the NHS. This is true, but it is not what the report means.

2 b. The report is insisting. It is saying that nurses have to be (are required to be) good communicators. Option **b** has this note. Although option **a** is true, it does not give the same impression.

3 a. Throughout the report the words 'there is a need for...' frequently appear. Because of the insistent note of the report, the words 'there is a need for' can be understood to mean 'there must be'.

4 c. In fact **a**, **b** and **c** are all true, but **c** is best because 'standards' involve both 'practices' and 'language'.

5 c. 'Access' is a flexible word and can refer to movement (option **a**). However, here 'access' is used as in 'I access my Emails', in other words, 'I get my Emails.' In the report, 'to have easy access to training schemes' means that training schemes should be available and it should be practically possible for nurses to go on them, have time off from work, etc.

6 c.

Exercise 2i

a. Standards of work are <u>affected</u> by poor communication. (Note the spelling of 'affected', and compare with 'effective'.)

b. A nurse needs to be a <u>competent</u> communicator.

c. A nurse needs an understanding of dialects, accents, idioms and <u>colloquialisms</u>.

d. Standards need to be <u>consistent</u>.

e. To demand language competence would be a <u>contravention</u> of European laws.

f. The number of people <u>applying</u> for jobs in the NHS is rising.

g. Training schemes need to be <u>accessible</u> to all newly recruited nurses.

Chapter Three

Nursing in the UK

Medical services are not organised in identical ways in every country so the following article gives an outline of the work of doctors and nurses in the UK.

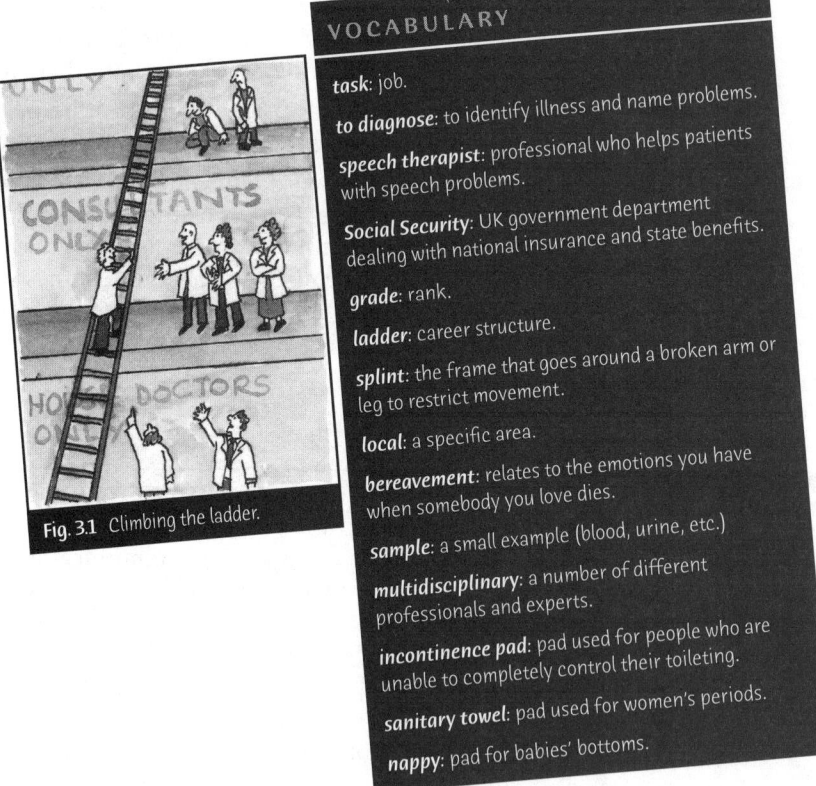

Fig. 3.1 Climbing the ladder.

VOCABULARY

task: job.

to diagnose: to identify illness and name problems.

speech therapist: professional who helps patients with speech problems.

Social Security: UK government department dealing with national insurance and state benefits.

grade: rank.

ladder: career structure.

splint: the frame that goes around a broken arm or leg to restrict movement.

local: a specific area.

bereavement: relates to the emotions you have when somebody you love dies.

sample: a small example (blood, urine, etc.)

multidisciplinary: a number of different professionals and experts.

incontinence pad: pad used for people who are unable to completely control their toileting.

sanitary towel: pad used for women's periods.

nappy: pad for babies' bottoms.

Doctors

The general practitioner (also known as the family doctor or GP) works from a surgery. The GP's main <u>task</u> is to <u>diagnose</u> and advise patients. The GP prescribes medicines, does minor surgery and refers patients to hospital specialists, social workers, psychologists, psychiatrists or <u>speech therapists</u>.

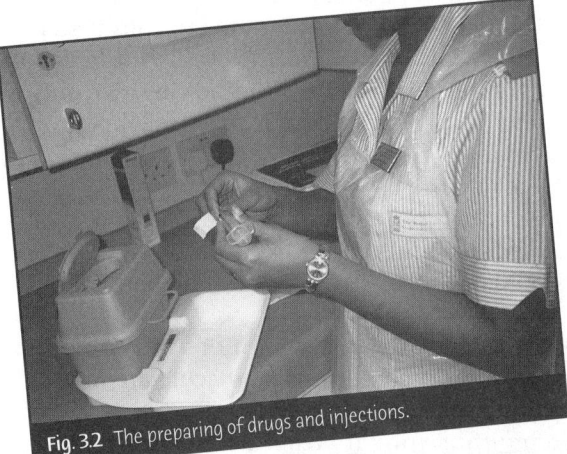
Fig. 3.2 The preparing of drugs and injections.

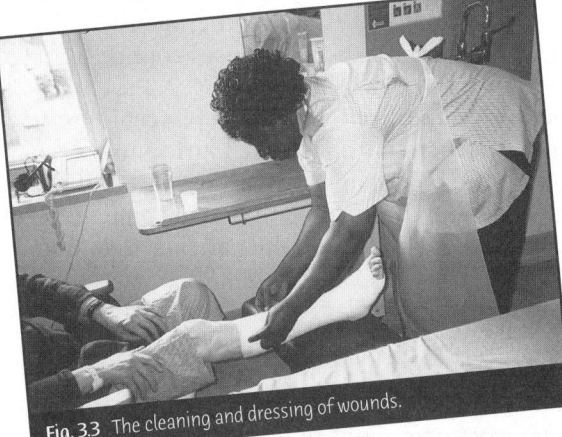
Fig. 3.3 The cleaning and dressing of wounds.

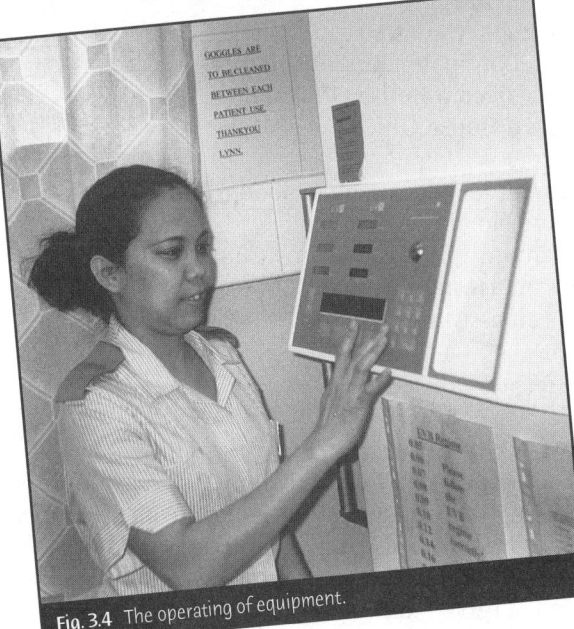
Fig. 3.4 The operating of equipment.

The GP also does things like certifying a patient's state of health for <u>Social Security</u> purposes, insurance companies and employers, and signing death certificates. The GP is involved in immunisation and checks on the development of babies. A big general practice not only employs doctors but also nurses, Health Visitors, Midwives and Physiotherapists.

There are several hospital doctor <u>grades</u>. A trainee doctor is known as a House Officer. The House Officer becomes a Senior House Officer and later a Specialist Registrar. At the top of the <u>hospital ladder</u> is the Consultant.

Nurses

A nurse's job is basically the same in the UK as it is everywhere. It includes:

- observing patients and assessing their responses to treatment.
- counselling patients and their relatives.
- taking temperatures, blood pressure and respiration rates.
- doing physical examinations.
- preparing instruments.
- administering drugs and injections.
- cleaning and dressing wounds.
- bandaging and <u>splinting</u>.
- administering blood transfusions and drips.
- preparing and handing instruments to surgeons in the operating theatre.
- operating equipment such as life-support systems and renal dialysis machines.

The Healthcare Assistant (also known as a Nursing Auxiliary) does the routine nursing tasks such as making beds and giving personal hygiene to patients confined to bed. A Registered Nurse does these tasks only for severely ill patients. The Healthcare Assistant is responsible for changing <u>incontinence pads, sanitary towels</u> and <u>nappies</u>, helping patients feed themselves, taking temperatures, checking pulse rates and respiration and noting them on reports.

A District Nurse is a nurse who visits people in their own homes or in residential care homes. A District Nurse trains patients to administer their own treatments.

Practice Nurses work in GPs' surgeries. They treat minor injuries and help with operations done under <u>local</u> anaesthetic. A Practice Nurse does health screening, family planning, <u>bereavement</u> counselling and immunisation, and gives advice to patients who want to give up smoking or lose weight. A Practice Nurse carries out investigations using electrocardiograms, gives hearing tests and takes blood <u>samples</u>. A Practice Nurse sometimes holds clinics for people with diabetes and asthma.

A Psychiatric Nurse works with patients with conditions including personality disorders, neuroses, phobic conditions, and acute anxiety, alcohol dependency, severe eating disorders and depression. A Psychiatric Nurse works in a <u>multidisciplinary team</u> with Psychiatrists, Clinical Psychologists, Health Visitors and Psychiatric Social Workers.

The Psychiatric Nurse's major role is to establish therapeutic relationships with patients. The Psychiatric Nurse uses counselling, group therapy, role-play, drama and discussion groups. A Psychiatric Nurse also gives patients drugs and injections. Seven per cent of nurses in the UK are men and many of them work as Psychiatric Nurses.

A Health Visitor is a nurse who works to *prevent* illness. A Health Visitor supports young mothers and their babies and visits patients with all kinds of chronic illnesses and disabilities in the patients' own homes.

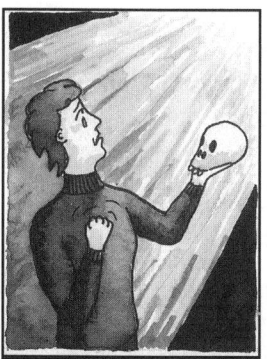

Fig. 3.5 A Psychiatric Nurse will employ drama and role-play in therapy.

Exercise 3a

Which of the following statements are true?

a. A GP is a doctor with a family.
b. A GP refers all patients who need operations to hospitals.
c. A GP refers patients who need operations to hospitals.
d. GPs are bureaucrats.
e. GPs deal with bureaucracy.
f. A House Officer is subordinate to a Consultant.
g. A Registrar will have been a House Officer.
h. A Registrar becomes a House Officer.
i. Nurses are councillors.
j. Only nurses who are qualified can give blood transfusions.
k. Only nurses can give blood transfusions.
l. Qualified nurses can only give blood transfusions.
m. A Practice Nurse is an assistant to a GP.
n. A Practice Nurse is an assistant GP.

Exercise 3b

Fill in the gaps in this text by using one word from each of the brackets:

Doctors .... (diagnose, prescribe, advise) medicines and nurses help .... (to administer, administer, administering) the treatment. Nurses .... (dress, operate, administer) sophisticated equipment, ... (take, give, bring) temperatures, blood pressures and respiration rates. They do not .... (give, administer, do) major operations but perform and............ (administer, assist, give) doctors with small operations .... (done to, done under, done by) local anaesthetic.

Exercise 3c

Complete the following sentences correctly:

a. Testing blood is usually .... by nurses.
b. A Practice Nurse will .... clinics for people with diabetes.
c. The Healthcare Assistant will .... incontinence pads, etc. as and when clean ones are necessary.
d. Patients' temperatures should be .... regularly.
e. We are going to .... out an investigation before operating.
f. A Health Visitor's main concern is in .... illness.
g. A Health Visitor's main concern is to .... illness.
h. A Practice Nurse's job includes .... advice to patients.

Exercise 3d

Choose the word or phrase (a, b, c or d) which best completes each of the following sentences:

The NHS versus private medicine

1 The NHS has a good .... for the treatment of chronic illnesses and research.
  a. record
  b. story
  c. account
  d. background

2 The NHS has greatly improved conditions for .... ill people and geriatrics.
  a. psychiatric
  b. mental
  c. mentally
  d. psychology

3 A national health service means equality of healthcare – each person is equally important .... his or her ability to pay.
  a. without regard
  b. regarding
  c. disregarding
  d. regardless of

4 With private health medicine, 'customers' can .... choices.
  a. do
  b. make
  c. take
  d. choose

5 Organisations like private hospitals that are run for profit are more efficient and waste .... money.
  a. fewer
  b. lesser
  c. less
  d. smaller

6 Some say it is wrong that richer people .... the best medical treatment.
  a. take

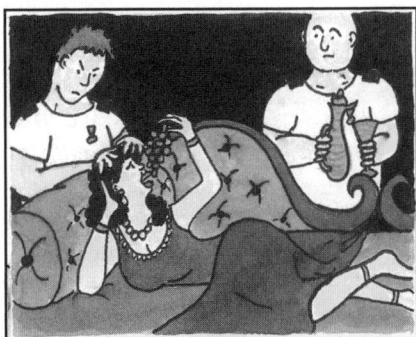
Fig. 3.6 Is it wrong that rich people can get the best health treatment?

  b. do
  c. get
  d. use

7 Private medicine can have low .... and there have been problems with 'cowboy' clinics.
  a. standards
  b. standard
  c. levels
  d. graded

8 In the past an NHS doctor could refer patients to any centres, now the patient .... where there is a contract.
  a. going
  b. is gone
  c. went
  d. goes

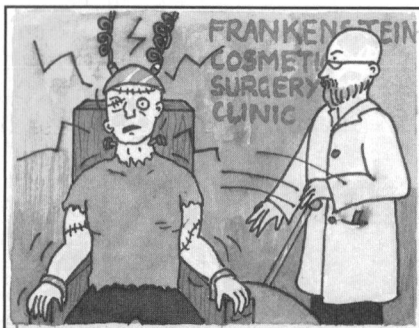

Fig. 3.7 Commercialising medicine can lead to low standards.

Exercise 3e

Put the correct form of the verb in brackets into the gaps in the following sentences. The first one is done as an example.

The nurse .... the patient's temperature an hour ago. (take)

<u>Answer:</u> The nurse <u>took</u> the patient's temperature an hour ago.

  a. Records of base-line functions must .... as accurately as possible. (make)
  b. The patient .... a blood transfusion on the 21st of last month. (give)
  c. Mr Hussein's wound should .... this morning but the nurse was interrupted and it wasn't done. (dress)
  d. A Bereavement Nurse was asked .... Mrs Dobson's relatives after she died. (counsel)
  e. It was necessary for the instruments to have .... in advance of the operation. (prepare)
  f. We would .... Mr Jameson to the County Hospital but we knew there were no beds available. (refer)
  g. The nurse was about .... an injection when the patient told her she was allergic to penicillin. (give)

Exercise 3f

Fill in the spaces in the following text about Nurse Practitioners with: in, up, for, to, since, on, during, from, with.

The idea of Nurse Practitioners was first developed .... the USA .... the 1970s and they have grown .... popularity in the UK .... the beginning of the 1990s. Though the RCN has defined the role of the Nurse Practitioner, it is not always clear whether a Nurse Practitioner is a mini-doctor or a maxi-nurse.

However, Nurse Practitioners are popular .... patients and many of them have moved .... primary healthcare .... hospitals as the idea has caught .... and it has become apparent that they both offer good value .... money and free .... medical time for doctors.

Health in the UK

A recent survey of the UK population has given us accurate information about the country's health. The information has important implications for the NHS.

There was a baby <u>boom</u> in the 1950s and 1960s in the UK and since then the birth rate has steadily <u>declined</u>. This means that the UK population is getting older. In fact it has the world's fifth highest population of older people. In Europe as a whole, the number of people over the age of 75 is projected to double over the next five years. The number of people over 90 years old will increase five-<u>fold</u>.

Now, for the first time ever, there are more people in the UK who are over 60 than under 16. The over-60s make up one-fifth of the population. The number of <u>centenarians</u> is also <u>set</u> to increase. In 1950 there were 300 and by the year 2030 there are expected to be 35 000. The number of over-85s has increased by 500% since 1951 and is now 1.1 million. The average <u>life-expectancy</u> has risen. Now it is 78 years for women and 74 years for men.

Care of the elderly takes up 40% of the NHS budget and it is a growing industry which employs over a million-and-a-half people.

The census has also provided the following information about the UK population:

- 156 people in every 1000 suffer from a neurotic <u>disorder</u>.
- 35 000 people die each year as a result of a brain-related disease.
- 10% of the population suffer from migraines.
- Myalgic encephalomyelitis (ME) affects about 2% of the population, which means 24 000 children in the UK have ME symptoms.
- Stroke is a leading cause of death and affects 1 in 500 people every year.
- 2 out of every 1000 babies born in the UK are affected by cerebral palsy. (There has been no change in this figure for the last 30 years.)
- Down's syndrome affects 1 in 1000 babies.
- 1 in 1000 babies in the UK is born with spina bifida.
- 1 in 4 people suffers from mental illness.
- 115 000 families are affected by autism. (Autism has a tendency to run in families.)
- 10% of autistic people excel as artists, mathematicians or musicians.
- 1 in 100 people suffers from dyslexia. Three times as many boys are dyslexic than girls.
- In the UK, 12 million people visiting their GP over one year will have symptoms of mental illness and 90 million working days are lost each year as a result of mental health problems.

Exercise 3g

The following sentences give some of the same information again but written in different ways. Use words from the text, alter them and add to them where necessary and use them to complete these sentences by putting them into the spaces.

a. The birth rate .... during the 1950s and 1960s. (Verb from 'boom')
b. Since then, the birth rate has been steadily .... (Meaning: falling in numbers)
c. The projection is that the number of Europeans over the age of 75 .... over the next five years. (Meaning: will increase by two times)
d. There has been a .... increase in the number of people over 85 years old since 1951. (Meaning: times five or 500%)
e. The average British woman can .... to live for 78 years. (Meaning: is able to anticipate/hope)
f. 10% of the population are migraine .... (Meaning: people who are affected by an illness)
g. Every year there are 35 000 .... through brain-related diseases. (Meaning: mortalities)
h. There is .... of 90 million working days each year because of mental illness. (Noun from 'lose')
i. There are .... people in 15 000 families in the UK. (Adjective from 'autism')
j. Soon the country will be .... by a majority of older people. (Verb from 'population')

Exercise 3h

Study the grammar of these expressions that are taken from the text above and then complete the sentences that follow them.

- 156 people in every 1000
- two out of every 1000
- (they) make up one-fifth of the (population)
- a five-fold increase
- the number has increased by 500%
- an increase in numbers
- one in 4
- three times as many

a. There will be .... two .... increase .... the number of people over the age of 75 years within five years.
b. There .... be twice .... many old people in the UK in five .... time.
c. The population of the UK is .... up .... more old people than young people.
d. .... of .... 1000 babies, 2 are born with cerebral palsy.
e. The number .... old people in the UK .... increase .... 200% in the next five years.
f. One in .... ten people suffers from migraines.
g. There has been .... 500% increase .... the number of over-85s.

Answers and comments on the language

Exercise 3a

a. is not true. A GP is a family doctor – a local doctor who sees all kinds of patients.

b. is not true. The text tells us that GPs may perform minor surgery themselves.

c. is true. If the sentence read 'A GP refers *all* patients...' then it would not be true.

d. is not true. A 'bureaucrat' is an administrator usually working for the government.

e. is true. 'Dealing with bureaucracy' means doing administrative tasks. 'To deal with' is 'to do', 'to handle', etc.

f. is true. 'Subordinate' means 'under', 'lower than' or 'taking orders from'.

g. is true. Note that 'will have been' tells us that a Registrar was a House Officer in the past but is no longer one.

h. is not true. The opposite is true, i.e. a House Officer becomes a Registrar.

i. is not true. Note the difference between a 'counsellor' who listens and perhaps gives advice (or counsels) and a 'councillor', who is an elected local government politician.

j. is true.

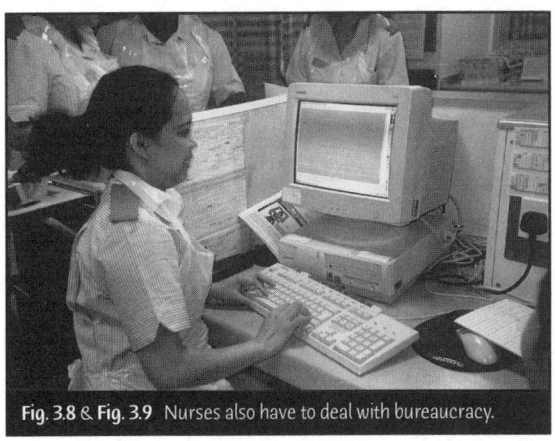
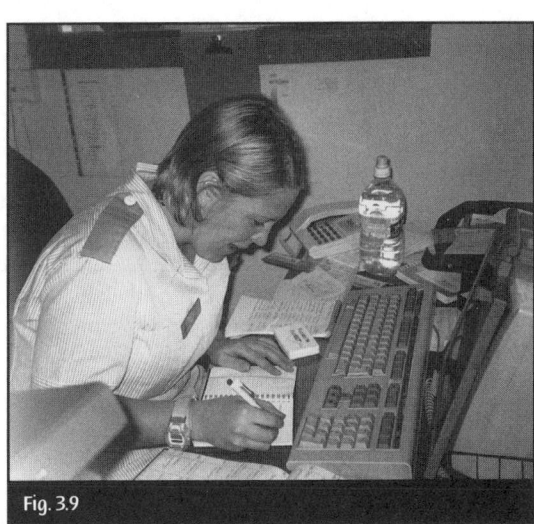

Fig. 3.8 & Fig. 3.9 Nurses also have to deal with bureaucracy.   **Fig. 3.9**

k. is not true. The position in the sentence of the word 'only' means that other people, like doctors for example, cannot give blood transfusions.

l. is not true. The sentence means that qualified nurses cannot do anything else but give blood transfusions.

m. is true.

n. is not true. An Assistant GP is a GP who assists, whereas 'an assistant to a GP' (question m) assists a GP.

Exercise 3b

Doctors <u>prescribe</u> medicines and nurses help to <u>administer</u> the treatment. Nurses <u>operate</u> sophisticated equipment, <u>take</u> temperatures, blood pressures and respiration rates, they do not <u>do</u> major operations but perform and <u>assist</u> doctors with small operations <u>done under</u> local anaesthetic.

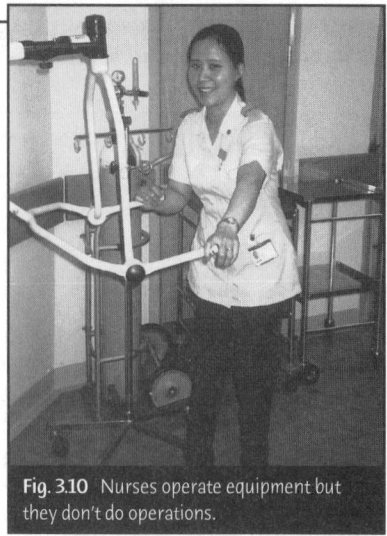

Fig. 3.10 Nurses operate equipment but they don't do operations.

Exercise 3c

a. Testing blood is usually <u>done</u> by nurses.
b. A Practice Nurse will <u>hold</u> clinics for people with diabetes.
c. The Healthcare Assistant will <u>change</u> incontinence pads, etc. as and when clean ones are necessary.
d. Patients' temperatures should be <u>taken/checked/measured/recorded</u> regularly.
e. We are going to <u>carry</u> out an investigation before the operation.
f. A Health Visitor's main concern is in <u>preventing</u> illness.
g. A Health Visitor' main concern is to <u>prevent</u> illness.
h. A Practice Nurse's job includes <u>giving/imparting</u> advice to patients.

Exercise 3d

1 The NHS has a good <u>record</u> for the treatment of chronic illnesses and research.

2 The NHS has greatly improved conditions for <u>mentally</u> ill people and geriatrics.

3 A national health service means equality of healthcare – each person is equally important <u>regardless</u> of his or her ability to pay.

4 With private medicine, 'customers' can <u>make</u> choices.

5 Organisations like private hospitals that are run for profit are more efficient and waste <u>less</u> money.

6 Some say it is wrong that richer people <u>get</u> the best medical treatment.

7 Private medicine can have low <u>standards</u> and there have been problems with 'cowboy' clinics.

8 In the past an NHS doctor could refer patients to any centres, now the patient <u>goes</u> where there is a contract.

Exercise 3e

a. Records of base-line functions must <u>be made</u> as accurately as possible. (make)

b. The patient <u>was given</u> a blood transfusion on the 21st of last month.

c. Mr Hussein's wound should <u>have been dressed</u> this morning but the nurse was interrupted and it wasn't done.

d. A Bereavement Nurse was asked <u>to counsel</u> Mrs Dobson's relatives after she died.

e. It was necessary for the instruments to have <u>been prepared</u> in advance of the operation.

f. We would <u>have referred</u> Mr Jameson to the County Hospital but we knew there were no beds available.

g. The nurse was about <u>to give</u> an injection when the patient told her she was allergic to penicillin.

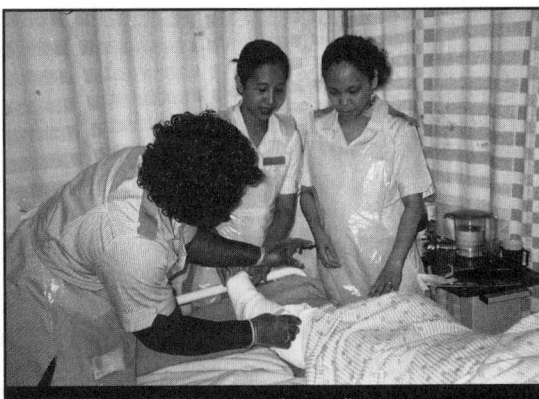

Fig. 3.11 'This should have been done earlier.'

Exercise 3f

The idea of Nurse Practitioners was first developed <u>in</u> the USA <u>in/during</u> the 1970s and they have grown <u>in</u> popularity in the UK <u>since</u> the beginning of the 1990s. Though the RCN has defined the role of the Nurse Practitioner, it is not always clear whether a Nurse Practitioner is a mini-doctor or a maxi-nurse.

However, Nurse Practitioners are popular <u>with</u> patients and many of them have moved <u>from</u> primary healthcare <u>into</u> hospitals as the idea has caught <u>on</u> and it has become apparent that they both offer good value <u>for</u> money and free <u>up</u> medical time for doctors.

Exercise 3g

a. The birth rate <u>boomed</u> during the 1950s and 1960s.
b. Since then, the birth rate has been steadily <u>declining</u>.
c. The projection is that the number of Europeans over the age of 75 <u>will</u> <u>double</u> over the next five years.
d. There has been a <u>five-fold</u> increase in the number of people over 85 years old since 1951.
e. The average British woman can <u>expect</u> to live for 78 years.
f. 10% of the population are migraine <u>sufferers</u>.
g. Every year there are 35 000 <u>deaths</u> through brain-related diseases.
h. There is <u>a loss</u> of 90 million working days each year because of mental illness.
i. There are <u>autistic</u> people in 15 000 families in the UK.
j. Soon the country will be <u>populated</u> by a majority of older people.

Exercise 3h

a. There will be <u>a</u> two-<u>fold</u> increase <u>in</u> the number of people over the age of 75 years within five years.
b. There <u>will</u> be twice <u>as</u> many old people in the UK in five <u>years'</u> time.
c. The population of the UK is <u>made</u> up <u>of</u> more old people than young people.
d. <u>Out</u> of <u>every</u> 1000 babies, 2 are born with cerebral palsy.
e. The number <u>of</u> old people in the UK <u>will</u> increase <u>by</u> 200% in the next five years.
f. One in <u>every</u> ten people suffers from migraines.
g. There has been <u>a</u> 500% increase <u>in</u> the number of over-85s.

Part Two

Records and notes

Chapter Four

The need for good records

Throughout this part of the book, you will be reading examples of nurses' notes and records, so the text that follows is *about* keeping notes and records. It is in the form of a memo addressed to the doctors, nurses and paramedics at a hospital in the UK from the hospital's Medical Director.

MEMO. TO ALL MEDICAL STAFF:
Guidance for taking notes and keeping records
FROM THE MEDICAL DIRECTOR.

A number of problems are occurring throughout the hospital because some staff are keeping <u>inaccurate and insufficient</u> records of observations, assessments and treatments.

I want to <u>draw the attention</u> of all staff to the importance of good record-keeping and ask everyone to read these guidelines.

Principles:

- Records primarily serve the interests of the patient.
- Records should be an accurate <u>chronology of events</u> – recording all consultations, assessments, observations, decisions and outcomes.
- Records are an essential means of communicating amongst staff.
- Records show that everyone has fulfilled his/her duty of care.

Practice:

- Use black ink to make photocopying easier.
- Write clearly and without spelling mistakes.
- Print your name underneath your signature.
- In your records highlight any <u>important abnormalities</u>.
- Use only abbreviations which are <u>in common use</u> in this hospital.
- Document all care as soon as it is given.
- If you think that a patient has been involved in an assault or self-harm, make a note of this to warn others.
- Record if the patient is <u>in the custody of the police</u>.
- Use rating scales to assess levels of pain, etc. which are in common use throughout the hospital.

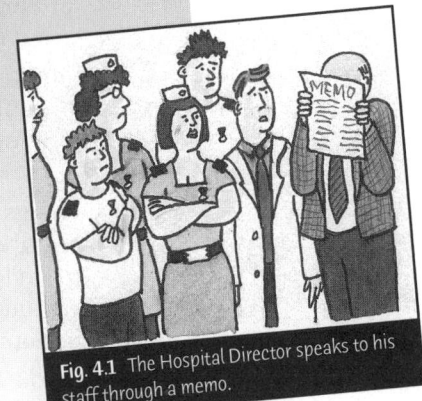

Fig. 4.1 The Hospital Director speaks to his staff through a memo.

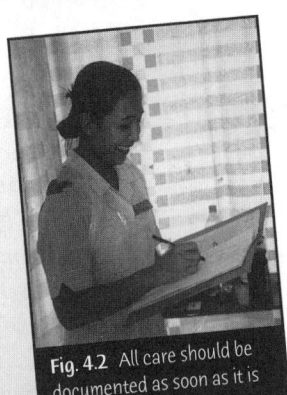

Fig. 4.2 All care should be documented as soon as it is given.

Exercise 4a

Practise using the vocabulary in the Medical Director's memo by answering the following questions:

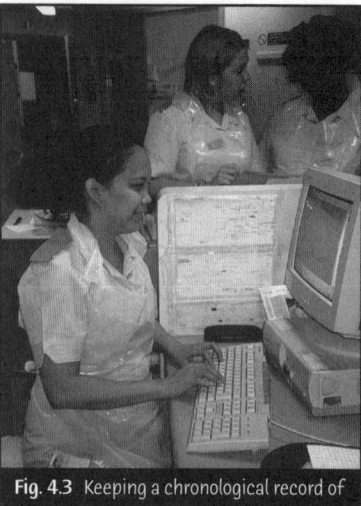

Fig. 4.3 Keeping a chronological record of events.

1   <u>inaccurate and insufficient</u> is closest in meaning to:
   a. bad and weak.
   b. wrong and not enough.
   c. unclear and too complicated.

2   To <u>draw the attention</u> is to:
   a. make a picture of the problem.
   b. highlight something.
   c. explain something.

3   A <u>chronology of events</u> is:
   a. a record of the important things.
   b. a record of the time when things happen.
   c. a record of how long it takes for each thing to happen.

4   <u>Important abnormalities</u> are:
   a. significant mistakes.
   b. relevant problems.
   c. the usual things.

5   Things that are <u>in common use</u> in the hospital are:
   a. only known by patients.
   b. understood by all staff.
   c. understood by laymen.
   d. popular.

6   If you are <u>in the custody of the police</u> you are:
   a. employed by the police.
   b. protected by a bodyguard.
   c. under arrest.

Exercise 4b

When writing, it is best, wherever possible, to use active, direct sentences rather than passive ones. To practise this, change these passive sentences into active ones. The first is done for you.

a. Many problems are created by poor records.
Answer: Poor records create many problems.

b. Everyone has been asked by the Medical Director to read the guidelines.
c. The interests of the patients are served by good records.
d. Black ink should be used by everyone.
e. All care should be immediately documented by nursing staff.
f. Levels of pain are described by rating scales.

Making notes and reading other people's notes

Medical forms and documents are not standardised in the UK – they vary between hospitals and even between departments in the same hospital.

Sometimes 'Nursing Instructions' are called 'Nursing Interventions'; sometimes 'Eating and Drinking' is called 'Food and Fluid Intake', sometimes 'Daily Living' is called 'Work and Play' and sometimes 'Aims and Objectives' are called 'Discharge Goals', 'Intended Goals', and so on.

Things like Patient Care Plans are usually hand-written, not typed, and usually written quickly by people in a hurry in short note form – not full sentences. Notes are not complete and 'good' English; they are full of abbreviations, arrows crossing the paper here and there, slashes, asterisks, stars, dots, underlinings, etc. Sometimes it is difficult to understand another person's notes – hard enough in your own language – extra difficult in a language not your own.

Sometimes medical abbreviations differ according to the field of healthcare. For example, POP is 'plaster of Paris' in Orthopaedics and 'posterior occipital position' in Midwifery.

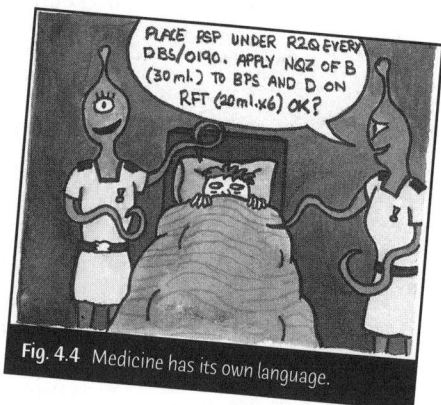

Fig. 4.4 Medicine has its own language.

Exercise 4c

These are notes on a 'Patient Care Plan'. Read them and answer the questions that follow:

Patient's problems	Goals	Nursing instructions
Poss. pressure sores due to poor skin. Because of arthritis & previous radiotherapy – general immobility	Healthy, intact skin	a. change position every 2 h, straighten sheets, remove crumbs (if any) use draw sheets. 2 nurses to turn patient b. personal hygiene – keep skin clean and dry. Assist with daily bedbath. N.B. hair & nails c. encourage nourishing diet with adequate protein and at least 2 l fluid

Problems

1 According to the notes, pressure sores may be caused by the patient's:
a. arthritis.
b. arthritis and radiotherapy.
c. inability to move.
d. dermatological problems.

2 The patient:
a. is having radiotherapy.
b. may have radiotherapy.
c. has had radiotherapy.

Goals

3 The nursing goals are to:
a. keep the patient's skin healthy.
b. get the patient's skin healthy.
c. get the patient healthy with skin intact.

Nursing Instructions

4 According to the 'Nursing Instructions', which of these statements are true? Nurses must:
a. change position every two hours.
b. move the patient every two hours.
c. help each other give the patient a bedbath.
d. help the patient give herself a bedbath.
e. keep their skin clean and dry.
f. not pay too much attention to the patient's hair and nails.

Exercise 4d

Here are the notes written out in full sentences. Complete the sentences by choosing one of the options in the brackets:

A ...... (mixing, number, combination) of arthritis and her recent radiotherapy has rendered the patient immobile. Consequently, the patient has poor ...... (skin, skins) and ...... (should, can, may) soon get pressure sores. Use two nurses to change the patient's position ...... (every, each, all) two hours. Use draw sheets and ...... (straight, straighter, straighten) them as well as ...... (removal, removed, removing) crumbs if there are any in her bed.

Her skin should be kept clean and dry and the patient should ...... (be having, have, had) a bedbath every day. Remember ...... (cleaning, clean, to clean) her hair and nails. She should be ...... (encouraged, encouraging, encourage) to eat a nourishing diet containing adequate protein and ...... (to drink, to be drinking, to have drunk) at least 2 litres of fluid ...... (all, every) day.

VOCABULARY

blemishes: marks on the skin.

discoloration: not the normal colour.

pubic area: genital area (covered by pubic hair.)

perineal (from 'perineum'): space between anus and scrotum.

disposable: equipment you throw away after using once.

after-effects: what happens afterwards.

abnormalities: things that are wrong (not normal).

Here is an extract from another Patient Care Plan. Study the vocabulary and read the extract carefully.

Goals	Nursing Instructions
Prevent pressure sores &/or cross-infection following catheterisation & reduce risk of ascending infection	Watch for blemishes, redness or discoloration & report. Wash, rinse & dry pubic area (use disposable) – washing from front of perineal area to back. Catheter care. Antiseptic cream to catheter. Monitor after-effects & report abnormalities.

Exercise 4e

Complete the following sentences using one of the choices provided:

1 The main goal is:
a. to eradicate infection.
b. to prepare the patient for catheterisation.
c. to avoid problems resulting from catheterisation.
d. to avoid problems resulting in catheterisation.

2 Nurses are instructed to:
a. watch how blemishes develop.
b. see whether blemishes develop.
c. observe when blemishes develop.

3 The patient's pubic area should be washed:
a. from back to front.
b. from front to rear.
c. only in the front.

4 The catheter is:
a. in danger…
b. dangerous…
c. endangered…
…of causing infection.

5 'Monitor after-effects' means:
a. Record the effects afterwards.
b. Watch for anything that happens after the catheterisation.
c. Make records after the patient has been catheterised.

Exercise 4f

Now the extract is written here in complete sentences. Fill the spaces in the sentences using the correct word from each of the brackets.

As you wash each part of the patient's body, observe .... (a, the, some) skin for .... (some, these, any) blemishes, ... (red, reddish, redness) or discoloration which could alert you to potential .... (develop, development, developed) of pressure sores. Wash, rinse and dry the patient's pubic .... (area, space, part) using disposables and wash .... (on, to, from) the front of the perineal area to the .... (back, reverse, after) in order .... (preventing, prevention, to prevent) cross-infection from the anal .... (space, district, region).

Carry .... (on, in, out) catheter care to help reduce the risk of ascending infection .... (via, towards, along with) the catheter to other parts of the .... (urine, urinating, urinary) system. Regularly .... (apply, application, applied) antiseptic cream to the catheter–urethra junction.

Patient records: the law

Anything that makes reference to a patient, such as a care plan or a diary, can be used as evidence in a law court. Care plans and diaries are used, for example, when investigating complaints of medical negligence or professional misconduct.

All medical staff have a legal duty to record care and this needs to be a full account of assessment, care planned and care provided. Entries in records must be frequent, especially when staff are presented with complex problems and deviations from the norm. It is particularly important to keep records if the condition of a patient does not appear to change, because a court of law will assume that if it is not recorded it has not been done.

The advantages of computer technology are that records are less bulky and there is less need for duplication. But the same principles of confidentiality apply to computer records as they do to manual ones. Any computer system that is used must be secure, any changes made to records should not make original entries disappear and anyone making an entry should be easily identifiable.

Patients do not have the right to limit the amount of information that goes in their records but they do have the right to limit access to them.

Exercise 4g

Say which of the following sentences are grammatically correct.

a. Care plans and diaries can be used as evidence.
b. Care plans and diaries are evidence.
c. A care plan is evidence.

d. Keep a record of care planned and care provided.
e. Keep records of care planning and provision.
f. Keep a record of care plan and provided.

g. Computer records are not so bulky.
h. Computer records are fewer bulky.
i. Computer records are decreased bulky.

j. An entry needs to be signature.
k. An entry needs a signature.
l. An entry needs signing.
m. An entry needs to be signed.

n. A patient cannot able to limit the amount of information.
o. A patient is not able limiting the amount of information.
p. A patient are not able to limit the amount of information.
q. No patient can limit the amount of information.

Exercise 4h

Here are extracts from the text 'Patient records: the law'. Say which of a, b and c means the same as each extract.

1 'Entries in records must be frequent.'
a. Make entries often.
b. Don't be long making entries.
c. Read the records regularly.

2 'Medical negligence'
a. Careless practice.
b. Neglected staff.
c. Attacks on patients.

3 'Professional misconduct'
a. A mistake.
b. An accident.
c. Bad behaviour.

4 'Deviations from the norm'
a. Predictable events.
b. Illegal incidents.
c. The unexpected.

5 'Confidentiality'
a. Secrecy.
b. Privacy.
c. Certainty.

6 'Any computer system that is used must be secure.'
a. Don't let anyone steal the computer.
b. Keep the computer in a safe place.
c. Access to data must be limited.

7 'Anyone making an entry must be easily identifiable.'
a. All entries must be signed.
b. You only have access to your own entries.
c. Identify yourself in order to get access to the records.

8 'Patients do have the right to limit access to their records.'
a. A patient has limited rights of access to their records.
b. A patient can say who can read their records and who can't.
c. Patients are correct to limit access to their records.

9 'There is less need for duplication.'

  a. We don't need a duplicator any more.

  b. There is not so much need to duplicate.

  c. Now we can make copies more easily.

Answers and comments on the language

Exercise 4a

1 b. It is difficult to predict whether the negative form of an English word uses the suffix in-, un- or non- (see Chapter 14, exercise 14c). There are three examples in this question: 'inaccurate', 'insufficient' and 'unclear'.

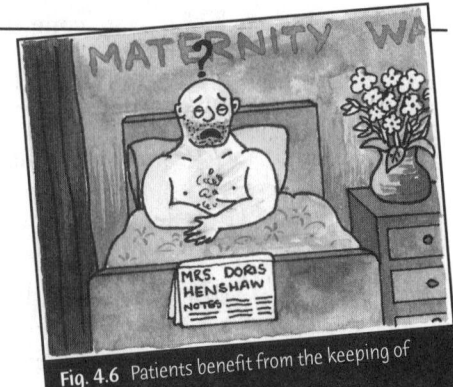

Fig. 4.5 Abnormalities in eating behaviour.

2 b. Often the verb 'to pay' goes with 'attention', but not always. Compare: 'I want you to pay attention to...' with, 'I want to draw your attention to...'

3 b. 'Chronology' is related to 'chronometer', which is an old word for 'clock'.

4 b. 'Abnormal' means 'not right' or 'not natural' or 'not healthy' and is frequently used in medical descriptions. For example, 'the child has abnormal eating habits'. This could mean that the child eats too much or too little or even that the child likes to eat glass!

5 b. Note the difference between 'common' and 'popular'. If something is popular, there is a suggestion that people like it as in: 'cannabis is popular with young people'. If something is 'common', people don't necessarily like it as in: 'Diabetes is common in India'. 'Lay men' are people who are not in a particular profession or field (like medicine). Another version is 'lay people'.

6 c. Note 'under' + 'arrest' and 'in' + 'custody'.

Exercise 4b

b. The Medical Director has asked everyone to read the guidelines.

c. Good records serve the interests of the patients.

d. Everyone should use black ink.

e. Nursing staff should immediately document all care, or: Nursing staff should document all care immediately.

f. Rating scales describe levels of pain.

Fig. 4.6 Patients benefit from the keeping of good records.

Exercise 4c

1   **d.** On the Patient Care Plan the abbreviation 'poss.' means: 'possible'. This is important because, according to the notes, the patient does not have pressure sores at the moment but is in danger of getting them. Note also the position of the dash (–) which points to the causes of the patient's poor skin. Similarly, the patient's immobility is because of arthritis and radiotherapy. 'Immobile' means 'unable to move'.

2   **c.** 'Previous radiotherapy' is past radiotherapy.

3   **b.** 'To get' here means 'to make' and it refers to an aim. 'To keep' means 'to maintain' and suggests that the patient's skin is already healthy. Both 'healthy and intact' refer to the patient's skin (indicated by the comma) so 'healthy' does not refer to the patient's general condition (option **c**).

4   **a.** is not true. 'Nurses must change position every two hours' refers to the nurses not the patients.

b. is true. There is a potential confusion here. 'Change the position of the patient' refers to how the patient is lying in bed. 'Move the patient' could mean 'move the patient to a different place'.

c. is not true. The word 'assist' in the Nursing Instructions means 'help the patient wash herself'.

d. is true.

e. is not true. 'Nurses must keep *their* skin clean and dry' refers to the nurses themselves.

f. is not true. 'N.B. hair and nails' means 'take special note of hair and nails – don't forget them.'

Exercise 4d

A <u>combination</u> of arthritis and her recent radiotherapy has rendered the patient immobile. Consequently, the patient has poor <u>skin</u> and <u>may</u> soon get pressure sores. Use two nurses to change the patient's position <u>every</u> two hours. Use draw sheets and <u>straighten</u> them as well as <u>removing</u> crumbs if there are any in her bed.

Her skin should be kept clean and dry and the patient should <u>have</u> a bedbath every day. Remember <u>to clean</u> her hair and nails. She should be <u>encouraged</u> to eat a nourishing diet containing adequate protein and <u>to drink</u> at least 2 litres of fluid <u>every</u> day.

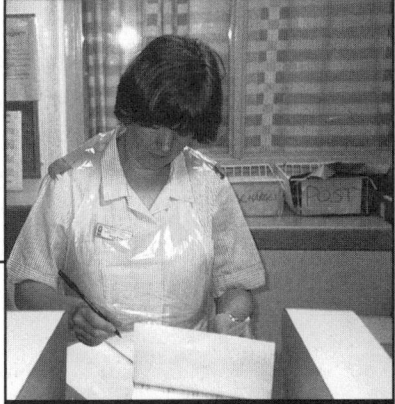

Fig. 4.7 Recording observations and care in a way everyone can understand.

Exercise 4e

1   **c.** At the moment there are no recorded problems on the sheet. The patient has been catheterised and there is a risk of infection, but as yet no visible infection.

2   b. 'Watch' + 'for' means 'be vigilant', 'be alert', etc. Both options **a** and **c** seem to assume that blemishes will develop but in fact we don't definitely know this.

3   b.

4   a. Note that if the '... of causing infection' part of the sentence had not been included, the correct sentence would have been, 'The catheter is dangerous.'

5   b.

Exercise 4f

As you wash each part of the patient's body, observe <u>the</u> skin for <u>any</u> blemishes, <u>redness</u> or discoloration which could alert you to potential <u>development</u> of pressure sores. Wash, rinse and dry the patient's pubic <u>area</u> using disposables and wash <u>from</u> the front of the perineal area to the <u>back</u> in order <u>to prevent</u> cross-infection from the anal <u>region</u>.

Carry <u>out</u> catheter care to help reduce the risk of ascending infection <u>via</u> the catheter to other parts of the <u>urinary</u> system. Regularly <u>apply</u> antiseptic cream to the catheter–urethra junction.

Exercise 4g

These sentences are grammatically correct:

a.
b.
c.
d.
e.
g.
k.
l.
m.
q.

Exercise 4h

1   a. Option **b** means 'make entries soon after doing something'.

2   a. Note that 'practice' means 'action' and 'routine' here.

3   c.

4   c. 'The norm' is the standard, the normal, expected thing. 'To deviate' is to move away from the standard, predictable thing.

5   b.

6   c.

7   a.

8   b. Note 'to have a right'. 'Rights' are legal and political notions – not to be confused with 'to be right' (option **c**).

9   b.

Chapter Five

Mrs Roberta Blackwood – attempted suicide

Read this description of a patient who was admitted to Accident and Emergency (A&E) when she took an overdose of paracetamol along with alcohol. Then read her A&E admission form which was completed when she arrived:

When Roberta Blackwood was admitted to A&E, she was sitting up, though she was a little <u>vague</u> and sleepy. She responded to verbal commands and was able to transfer herself from the ambulance trolley to the casualty trolley.

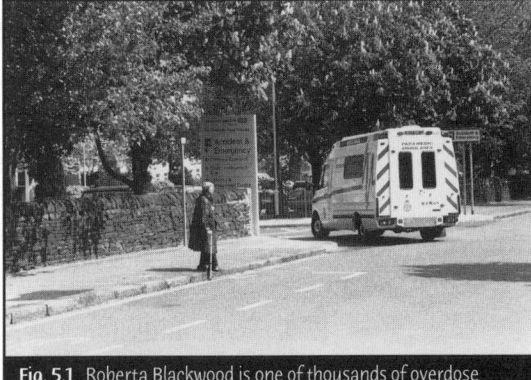

Fig. 5.1 Roberta Blackwood is one of thousands of overdose patients brought in to A & E each year.

Roberta's breath smelt of alcohol. However, there were no signs that she had vomited. Base-line functions were recorded on the admission form thus:

Base-line functions		
Breathing	Rate	Cough
	16/min	nil
Circulation	Pulse rate	BP
	92/min	105/65 mmHg
Colour	Skin	Lips
	OK	pink
Eyes		
Pupils react to light OK		

Roberta was accompanied in the ambulance by her aunt, Mrs Judith Smart. The patient had telephoned her aunt an hour earlier telling her what she had done and asking her to take care of her baby.

At the time the admission form was completed, Roberta was very withdrawn, avoided looking at people and would not speak. Later, however, after some counselling by an A&E staff nurse, she began to talk more openly.

Roberta has a baby. She is unskilled and unqualified and her husband works as a labourer. Roberta often visits a local pub with her aunt, who is her best friend. Her husband is out most evenings and when he returns, she says, he is usually drunk and often aggressive. She dreads her husband coming home at night but, though he is fairly rough with her, he has not beaten her up.

Roberta said she felt unable to cope with the situation at home. She said that the baby cried a lot and was very demanding and that she was not getting much sleep. Roberta is very anxious about the involvement of the Social Services and worries in case they will take her baby away.

Her parents arrived soon after she did and her father showed he was irritated at his daughter's actions. Her husband so far has not visited.

Exercise 5a

1 On admission, the patient was:
a. unconscious.
b. conscious and alert.
c. awake but drowsy.

2 On admission, the patient:
a. had been sick.
b. had not been sick.
c. was sick.

3 The patient:
a. came alone.
b. came with her baby.
c. came with a relative.

4 Her base-line functions show that the patient:
a. is not coughing.
b. cannot cough.
c. has no cough.

5 The patient is:
a. worried about the Social Services.
b. anxious to see someone from Social Services.
c. worried for the Social Services.

6 The patient's father is:
a. sympathetic.
b. indifferent.
c. antagonistic.

7 The patient says:
a. she has too much.
b. there's too much for her.
c. things are too much for her.

PATIENT ASSESSMENT RECORD

Name:
Roberta Blackwood

Prefers to be addressed as: Robbie

Address:
14 Hardcastle Terrace, Chesterton

Other persons important to patient:
husband: James

Whom to contact in emergency:
as above

DOB: 20.7.80   **Tel:** 0112 765432

Doctor:
Dr Sullivan

Primary nurse:
RSN Jane Smallweed

Reason for admission:
overdose – 25 paracetamol tabs (approx.) + gin.

Patient's understanding of admission:
patient embarrassed by admission – unresponsive but not unco-operative.

Source of assessment:
patient/aunt (Judith Smart) accompanying.

Family's understanding of admission:
husband & parents informed.

Drugs taken at home:
admits to use of cannabis (to help sleep)

MEDICAL INFORMATION

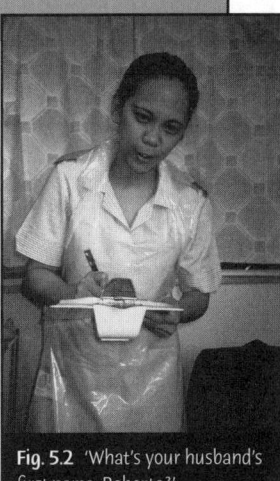

Fig. 5.2 'What's your husband's first name, Roberta?'

Relevant medical history
Feeling depressed/weepy over period, has baby 3 months – c/o aunt – consulted GP – no medication prescribed.

Medical diagnosis:
risk of hepatic failure due to ingestion of 12.5 g paracetamol/risk of respiratory depression due to drinking unknown amount alcohol.

Allergies:
penicillin

Patient's feelings and expectations related to present illness:
Patient is aware of dangers & poss. risks & will co-operate with stomach wash-out.

Nurse's initial impression (physical and social):
Patient is conscious but drowsy, uncommunicative & avoids eye contact, poss. poor relationship with husband (reported by aunt) – says, 'unable to cope with new baby'.
Attractive, slim young woman – not dirty or untidy.

Exercise 5b

Which of the following statements are <u>definitely</u> true at the time this Patient Assessment Record is completed? (Some statements may be true but you don't know for sure.)

a. Robbie is the patient's husband.
b. The patient was given too many paracetamol.
c. The patient is out cold.
d. The patient is violent.
e. Information comes from the patient's aunt.
f. The patient is unhappily married.
g. The husband knows about his wife's admission.
h. Robbie uses unprescribed drugs.
i. The patient has been to see her family doctor.
j. No one is available to take care of the baby.
k. The overdose will cause respiratory depression.

Exercise 5c

The following is part of Roberta Blackwood's Patient Assessment Record written out in full sentences. Put these words into the gaps in the text (some of them can be used more than once): at, to, in, on, of, ago, any, some, about, since, with, though.

Roberta Blackwood took an overdose .... 25 paracetamol and drank .... gin. She did not respond .... staff .... first but later spoke .... her problems .... home. She had a baby three months .... and has been feeling depressed .... then. She is not getting ...... with her husband and she says she is unable to cope .... the new baby.

She uses cannabis .... help her sleep and .... she has been in touch with her GP he did not prescribe .... medication. Roberta has agreed ...... co-operate with staff over a stomach wash-out because she understands the danger she is ....

Exercise 5d

The following sentences are taken from Roberta Blackwood's Patient Assessment Record. Choose, from a, b and c, which is the nearest in meaning to the underlined phrase:

1   Reason for admission
'The patient has overdosed on 25 paracetamol tablets <u>and an unknown quantity of alcohol</u>.'

a. The patient didn't know she was drinking alcohol.
b. Hospital staff don't know how much she has drunk.
c. The patient has mixed her drinks and so staff don't know exactly what she has been drinking.

2   Patient's understanding of admission
'<u>The patient is embarrassed by her admission</u>.'

a. The patient is embarrassing.
b. The patient is shy.
c. The patient is ashamed of herself.

3   Medical diagnosis
'<u>There is a risk of hepatic failure</u> due to the ingestion of 12.5 g of paracetamol.'

a. There is a danger that the liver will malfunction.
b. Liver failure creates risks.
c. A failed liver is dangerous.

4   Relevant medical history
'<u>The patient has been feeling depressed and weepy over a period of time.</u>'

a. The patient occasionally feels depressed.
b. She has always been depressed.
c. The patient has been feeling depressed for a while.

5   Nurse's initial impression
'<u>The patient is conscious but drowsy.</u>'

a. The patient is sleepy.
b. The patient is asleep.
c. The patient is unaware of anything.

Exercise 5e

Read the following article which reports on research linking an increase in attempted suicides with the accident which killed Princess Diana. Fill in the spaces with the correct word from each of the brackets.

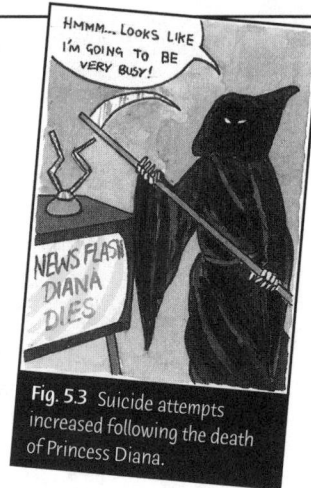

Fig. 5.3 Suicide attempts increased following the death of Princess Diana.

The death of Princess Diana and a rise in the suicide rate

Recent research by Professor Keith Hawton of Oxford University shows that the amount of suicide .... (attempting, attempted, attempts) by women in the UK increased dramatically .... (immediate, immediately) after the death of Princess Diana on 31st August 1997.

There was a 33.7% rise .... (at, on, in) suicides during the week following the accident, and a 65.1% rise .... (at, on, in) deliberate self-harm and .... (attempted, attempts, attempting) suicide.

There is a theory that an event like Diana's .... (die, died, death) brings people closer together with a shared sense of .... (sorry, sorrow) and that this social cohesion prevents any sudden .. .. (increased, increasing, increase) in suicide attempts. But not so in this case. Diana's death seemed to serve as a ... . (go, switch, trigger) for those who wanted ... . (to take, taking, took) their own lives.

According to Professor Hawton, 'Women related to Diana through the . ... (stressful, stressed out, stresses) and strains they saw in her life and some thought "Here was a young woman who had everything going .... (for, by, with) her and so what's the point in me .... (life, living, alive) when you could go just like that at .... (some, all, any) time?"'

Another cause of the .... (raise, risen, rise) in suicides, according to the research, is the .... (guilt, guilty) which people felt when Diana .... (died, death, dying). People felt responsible because they were part of the society which wanted to know about her and bought the newspapers and magazines which chased her. 'If it hadn't been for us,' people thought, 'she would not .... (be speeding, speeded, have been speeding) away in that car from press and cameramen.'

A spokeswoman for the Samaritans agreed with Professor Hawton but added, 'we wouldn't say her death .... (causing, cause, caused) anyone to kill themselves – it is never anyone .... (else's, else, else is) fault when someone takes .... (a, my, their) own life.'

Exercise 5f

Look at the following information about overdoses of paracetamol. Re-write each of the sentences so that they start with the words that are underlined. (The first is done for you as an example.)

1 It has been estimated by researchers that the NHS has 110 000 cases of overdose each year.

Researchers estimate ...

Answer: <u>Researchers estimate</u> that the NHS has 110 000 cases of overdose each year.

2   Less than one-quarter of all overdose patients intended to kill themselves.
<u>The majority of overdose patients</u> ...

3   Total medical admissions are made up of 14% overdoses.
<u>Overdoses make up</u> ...

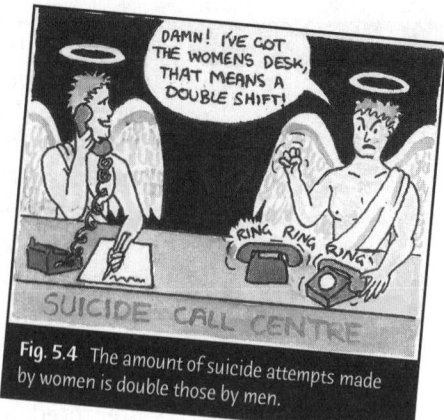

Fig. 5.4 *The amount of suicide attempts made by women is double those by men.*

4   Alcohol is taken by 25% of parasuicides.
<u>25%</u> ...

5   Suicide attempts are carried out by twice as many women as men.
<u>Women carry out</u> ...

6   40% of parasuicides use paracetamol.
<u>Paracetamol</u> ...

7   Hepatotoxicity and possible death can be caused by as few as 20 tablets (10 g) of paracetamol.
<u>As few as</u> ...

8   A stomach wash-out is recommended by doctors for overdoses of 20 tablets or more.
<u>Doctors</u> ...

9   Alcohol is also removed by the stomach wash-out.
<u>The stomach wash-out also</u> ...

10   Patients are not 'taught a lesson' by stomach wash-outs.
<u>Stomach wash-outs</u> ...

Suicide: the statistics

The UK has one of the highest suicide rates amongst European countries. In the UK and Ireland, approximately 6300 people kill themselves every year. This figure is double the rate for road traffic accidents and twelve times the rate for murders. This means that there is one suicide every 84 minutes. Twenty-six per cent of British people know someone who has killed themselves.

About 140 000 people attempt suicide every year and the trend is rising.

In 1994, there were 785 suicides by young people. This is about 2 per day.

If you look at suicide in terms of occupation, then the highest risk occupation for men is vets, who are three-and-a-half times more likely to kill themselves than the average person. The risk for dentists is just over twice the average, as it is for farmers and pharmacists.

Amongst women, the highest risk occupation is government inspector, which has a risk of four-and-a-half times the average. The second highest is vets, followed closely by medical practitioners, pharmacists, physiotherapists, ambulance women and other health professionals. Nurses are at 1.54 times the average risk and account for 5% of all female suicides between 1982 and 1992.

The view is that people use a method of suicide to which they have easiest access, so the most common method of suicide by both men and women in the health professions is self-poisoning because these people can get hold of drugs without any great difficulty. There has been an enormous increase in the use of paracetamol for suicide attempts over the past 20 years.

Relationship problems are most commonly associated with attempted suicide and it is very common for a serious argument with a partner to have happened just before a suicide attempt. Problems with a partner are more often mentioned by men who have attempted suicide than by women.

Other factors associated with suicide are unemployment, social deprivation, a history of physical or sexual abuse, alcohol problems and social isolation.

Repetitions of suicide attempts are common and 20% of people who attempt suicide are readmitted to hospital for the same reason within a year.

Exercise 5g

According to the information above, say which of the following statements are true:

a. More people die on the roads than commit suicide.
b. There are approximately twelve murders every year in the UK.
c. More than one-quarter of the population of the UK know someone who has killed themselves.
d. More vets kill themselves than any other occupational group.
e. Five out of a hundred nurses kill themselves.

Exercise 5h

Say which of these sentences are grammatically correct:

a. In 1994, 785 young people suicided.
b. 6300 people suicide themselves every year.
c. Poisoning of self is the most common method.
d. Self-poisoning is the most common method.
e. Relationship problems are the most common associated with suicide.
f. Repeat suicide attempts are not uncommon.
g. Suicide attempts to repeat are not uncommon.
h. There has been an increased use of paracetamol in suicide attempts.
i. Paracetamol is increasingly used in attempted suicides.
j. Paracetamol is increased use in attempted suicide.
k. Paracetamol is in increased use in attempted suicide.

Answers and comments on the language

Exercise 5a

1   c. 'Drowsy' means 'sleepy'. To drowse is to have a light sleep. 'Alert' (option **b**) means 'conscious and paying close attention to everything'.

2   b. 'to be sick' here means 'to vomit'. In other cases, it means 'to be ill'. For example, 'the patient is very sick' means the same as 'the patient is very ill.' 'Poorly' can mean the same as this meaning of 'sick', e.g. 'the patient is poorly.' The adjective 'sickly' means 'weak and prone to illness'. 'On admission the patient was sick' (option **c**) means 'the patient vomited at the time she was admitted'.

3   c. The words 'accompanied by' in the text mean that somebody went with Roberta to the hospital.

4   c. 'The patient has no cough' refers to regular coughing – as with smokers. Although option **c** is the best choice here, option **a** is also possible.

5   a. The text tells us that Roberta is 'anxious *about*' the Social Services. This means she is afraid of them. She is 'anxious *for* her baby'. This means she is 'worried about her baby' or 'worried for her baby'. 'Anxious to see someone from Social Services' (option **b**) means that she wants to see someone from Social Services whereas in fact the opposite is true.

6   c. 'Indifferent' (option **b**) means to not care/ to feel nothing about something. According to the text, the patient's father is 'irritated', which tells us that he does feel something even though it is not sympathy. 'Antagonistic' means 'hostile', 'angry', etc.

7   c. When 'things are too much' for you, you cannot 'cope with' or 'handle' life. Options **a** and **b** both mean that Roberta has a lot (not problems, but gifts perhaps).

Exercise 5b

a. is not true. 'Robbie' is the patient herself. 'Robbie' is a pet name or nickname. The term 'prefers to be addressed as' refers to the patient's preferred name and has nothing to do with where she lives (her address).

b. is not true. She was not 'given' them, she 'took' them.

c. is not true. 'Out cold' means unconscious and in fact the patient is described as 'conscious but drowsy'.

d. is not true. The patient is described as 'co-operative'.

e. is true. 'Information' rather than 'the information' means 'some' of the information.

f. is true. However, because the information comes second-hand from the patient's aunt, Roberta's marriage difficulties are described as 'poss. (possible) poor relationship with husband (reported by aunt).'

g. is true. Her husband has been informed (See: 'Family's understanding of admission').

h. is true. Cannabis is not prescribed to aid sleep.

i. is true. In 'Relevant medical history', we read that Roberta has consulted her GP.

j. is not true. The baby is in the care of Roberta's aunt. 'c/o…' means 'in the care of…'.

k. is not true. The words 'risk of' are used to describe a danger which is not yet a fact.

Exercise 5c

Roberta Blackwood took an overdose <u>of</u> 25 paracetamol and drank <u>some</u> gin. She did not respond <u>to</u> staff <u>at</u> first but later spoke <u>about</u> her problems <u>at</u> home. She had a baby three months <u>ago</u> and has been feeling depressed <u>since</u> then. She is not getting <u>on</u> with her husband and she says she is unable to cope <u>with</u> the new baby. She uses cannabis <u>to</u> help her sleep and, <u>although</u> she has been in touch with her GP, he did not prescribe <u>any</u> medication. Roberta has agreed <u>to</u> co-operate with staff over a stomach wash-out because she understands the danger she is <u>in</u>.

Exercise 5d

1 b.

2 c. Be careful about the differences between 'embarrassing' and 'embarrassed'. Similarly, people often mix up: 'boring' with 'bored' and 'frightened' with 'frightening'.

3 a.

4 c. Note that 'for a while' means a moderately long period. Option a – 'occasionally feels depressed' – means 'sometimes she feels depressed and sometimes she doesn't.'

5 a. Note that 'sleepy' does not mean 'asleep' but 'wants to sleep' or 'is trying to fully wake up after being asleep'. If the patient is 'unaware of anything' (option c) she would be unconscious or in some way cut off from the world around her.

Exercise 5e

The death of Diana and a rise in the suicide rate

Recent research by Professor Keith Hawton of Oxford University shows that the amount of suicide <u>attempts</u> by women in the UK increased dramatically <u>immediately</u> after the death of Princess Diana on 31st August 1997.

There was a 33.7% rise <u>in</u> suicides during the week following the accident, and a 65.1% rise <u>in</u> deliberate self-harm and <u>attempted</u> suicide. There is a theory that an event like Diana's <u>death</u> brings people closer together with a shared sense of <u>sorrow</u> and that this social cohesion prevents any sudden <u>increase</u> in suicide attempts. But not so in this case. Diana's death seemed to serve as a <u>trigger</u> for those who wanted <u>to take</u> their own lives.

According to Professor Hawton, 'Women related to Diana through the <u>stresses</u> and strains they saw in her life and some thought "Here was a young woman who had everything going <u>for</u> her and so what's the point in me <u>living</u> when you could go just like that at <u>any</u> time?"'

Another cause of the <u>rise</u> in suicides, according to the research, is the <u>guilt</u> which people felt when Diana <u>died</u>. People felt responsible because they were part of the society which wanted to know about her and bought the newspapers and magazines which chased her. 'If it hadn't been for us,' people thought, 'she would not <u>have been speeding</u> away in that car from press and cameramen.'

A spokeswoman for the Samaritans agreed with Professor Hawton but added, 'we wouldn't say her death <u>caused</u> anyone to kill themselves – it is never anyone <u>else's</u> fault when someone takes <u>their</u> own life.'

Exercise 5f

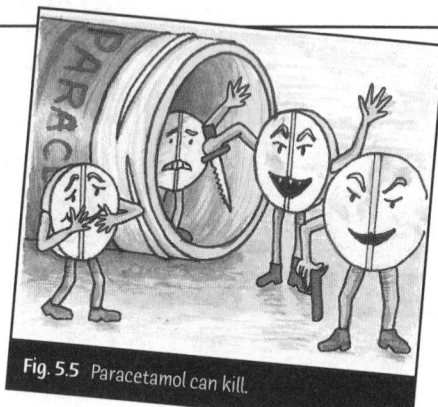

Fig. 5.5 *Paracetamol can kill.*

2 <u>The majority of overdose patients</u> do not intend to kill themselves.

3 <u>Overdoses make up</u> 14% of total medical admissions.

4 <u>25%</u> of parasuicides have taken/take alcohol.

5 <u>Women carry out</u> twice as many suicide attempts as men.

6 <u>Paracetamol</u> is used by 40% of parasuicides.

7 <u>As few as</u> 20 tablets of paracetamol can cause hepatotoxicity and death.

8 <u>Doctors</u> recommend a stomach wash-out for overdoses of 20 tablets or more.

9 <u>The stomach wash-out</u> also removes the alcohol.

10 <u>Stomach wash-outs</u> do not 'teach patients a lesson'.

Exercise 5g

a. is not true. The text tells us that there are twice as many suicides as road deaths.
b. is not true. There are twelve times as many suicides as murders.
c. is true.
d. is not true. When linking suicide with occupations, the text refers to *proportionate* risks. There are fewer vets than bus drivers, for example, and perhaps more bus drivers kill themselves than vets, but a higher proportion of the total amount of vets kill themselves than bus drivers.
e. is not true. Out of the total amount of female suicides, 5 out of 100 are nurses.

Exercise 5h

The following sentences are grammatically correct:

c.
d.
f.
h.
i.
k.

Chapter Six

Ms Ethel Partridge – diabetes

A young woman is admitted unconscious to hospital. This is her assessment record:

PATIENT ASSESSMENT RECORD

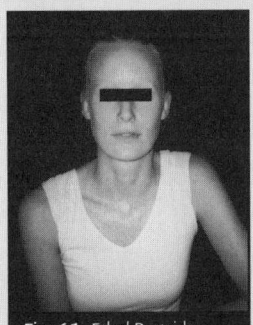

Fig. 6.1 Ethel Partridge. Born 1975. Diabetic.

Other persons important to patient:
Robert Greene (live-in partner)

DOB: 12.3.75

Tel. 01765 342189

Doctor:
Dr Sullivan

Primary nurse:
Jean Bradshaw

Name:
Ethel Partridge

Prefers to be addressed as: Effie

Address:
33 Madison Way, Lower Stockton

Whom to contact in emergency:
parents and Robert Greene

Reason for admission:
became unconscious after feeling unwell & increasingly drowsy

Patient's understanding of admission:
unconsciousness on admission

Source of assessment:
partner

Family's understanding of admission:
diabetes

Drugs taken at home:
contraceptive pill

MEDICAL INFORMATION

Relevant medical history:
nil

Medical diagnosis:
diabetic ketoacidosis

Allergies:
Elastoplast

Patient's feelings and expectations related to present illness:
unable to assess due to unconsciousness

Nurse's initial impression (physical and social):
physically fit, well-adjusted young woman with lots of friends

Knowledge/information/skills needed for continued self-care after discharge:
1. Diabetes and how it affects the body
2. Insulin therapy and self-administration
3. Factors affecting body's need for glucose

Exercise 6a

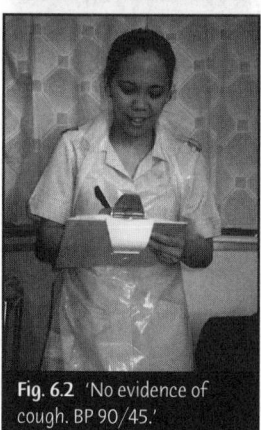

Fig. 6.2 'No evidence of cough. BP 90/45.'

Which of the following statements are true?

a. The patient's nickname is Ethel.
b. The patient is not married.
c. The patient's parents would not be able to get to the hospital in an emergency.
d. Jean Bradshaw is the head nurse of the hospital.
e. The patient was uncommunicative on admission.
f. The patient felt sleepy before falling unconscious.
g. The hospital got the information for the assessment form from the patient's parents.
h. The patient is diabetic.
i. The patient is diabetic ketoacidosis.
j. The patient has diabetes.

Exercise 6b

Read the next part of the Patient Assessment Form and use the information to complete the text that follows:

Base-line functions		
Breathing	**Rate**	**Cough**
	32/min	nil
Circulation	**Pulse rate**	**BP**
	128/min	90/45 mmHg
Colour	**Skin**	**Lips**
	pink	pink

Oral likes, dislikes, food intake   (Type, time regular appetite)
Likes   tea, coffee, wine
Dislikes   milk
Patient is: Thin/obese, (normal)
Teeth   Mouth
Own   clean & dry

The patient's breathing is ...... (on, in, at) a rate of 32 per minute and she does not ...... (to cough, coughing, have a cough). Her pulse rate ...... (are, to be, is) 128 per minute and her blood pressure is ...... (ninety times forty-five, ninety over forty-five, forty-five under ninety). She is ...... (at, in, of) normal body size and has ...... (owns teeth, all teeth, her own teeth.) She likes most drinks but ...... (dislike, dislikes, has a dislike) of milk.

Exercise 6c

Put: by, for, of, between, from, about, in, to, of, or as in the spaces in the following text:

When Ethel Partridge was admitted .... A&E, she was accompanied .... Mr Robert Greene who lives with her. They came .... ambulance and Mr Greene reported .... staff that his girlfriend had become sleepy, felt generally poorly and then fallen unconscious.

Ethel Partridge is diabetic and will require the supervision .... a diabetic nurse specialist in order .... learn how .... maintain metabolic control .... the future. She will need to know .... the brain's need .... glucose .... a source of fuel, the dangers .... hypoglycaemia resulting .... too much insulin relative .... food intake, the relationship .... stress and blood sugar levels and methods of testing urine .... ketones and blood .... sugar.

She needs to know how hyperglycaemia is related .... excessive food intake or eating the wrong kinds .... food, decreased activity levels .... relation .... food intake, illness and infections.

Exercise 6d

Here are questions about diabetes which someone like Ethel Partridge might ask. Complete both the questions and answers so that they are all grammatically correct by choosing an option from the brackets.

1   *Question*: Diabetics can't eat sweets .... (can they? do they? can't they?)
Answer: Sweets are .... (no worse, not less, not bad) for diabetics than other people.

2   *Question*: It isn't safe for diabetics to drive .... (are they? is it? doesn't it?)
Answer: Other people are .... (none safer, no safer, not safe) than diabetics.

3   *Question*: .... (Doesn't, Isn't, Aren't) too much sugar cause diabetes?
Answer: No, it's .... (a cause, causing, caused) by a combination of things – genes and environment.

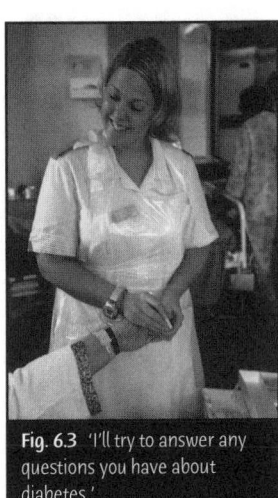

4   *Question:* .... (Don't, Doesn't, Aren't) people with diabetes eventually go blind?
Answer: It's possible, but it's .... (lesser, decreased, less) likely if you properly control blood pressure and glucose levels.

5   *Question:* .... (Won't it, Will it, Is it) possible to catch diabetes from another person?
Answer: No, we don't know why some people get it, but it .... (won't be, are not, isn't) contagious.

Fig. 6.3 'I'll try to answer any questions you have about diabetes.'

Exercise 6e

Read the following text about diabetes and fill in the gaps with the correct choice of word(s) from the brackets:

.... (Diabetes, Diabetics) was first recorded in .... (old, antique, ancient) Egypt in 1500 BC. The word 'diabetes' ...... (are, is, were) Greek and means 'fountain' referring to the large amounts of .... (urination, urine, urinary) produced by the disease in its .... (early, young, beginnings) stages. .... (Diabetes, Diabetic, A diabetic) urine smells sweet and its alternative name – 'mellitus' .... (come, comes, goes) from the Latin word for 'honey'. Doctors can often .... (found, finding, find) unsuspected diabetes by .... (find, found, finding) sugar in routine urine tests. The urine of diabetics attracts ants .... (look, looked, looking) for sugar and early methods of .... (detection, detect, detecting) diabetes included .... (taste, tasted, tasting) the urine for .... (sweet, sweeten, sweetness).

Exercise 6f

Ethel Partridge may need to be shown how to give herself injections of insulin. The following sentences are step-by-step instructions with key verbs left out. Using the list of verbs below, fill in the spaces in the instructions.

1   .... a needle and syringe of the correct size, making sure that they both remain aseptic and .... the needle on to the syringe.

2   The needle is .... through the rubber stopper of the medication bottle.

3   The prescribed dose of the fluid should be .... from the container into the syringe.

4   .... the bottle and syringe .... and pull back on the plunger to the required dosage of fluid.

5   .... the skin at the site chosen for the injection.

6   The syringe needs to be .... for air bubbles.

7   Using the hand you write with, hold the syringe like a pen or pencil and with the other hand .... about 2 to 3 inches on either side of the skin.

8   About ⅔ of the needle is .... at a 90° angle.

9   .... the piston of the syringe.

10   Pull the needle out smoothly and quickly and then .... of it.

VERBS

to assemble: to put together and prepare.

to pinch: to take a piece of skin between finger and thumb.

to turn upside down: to turn so that the top is underneath.

to insert: to put in.

to depress: to push down.

to dispose of: to get rid of/throw away.

to check: to look carefully and make sure.

to swab: to clean with alcohol saturated cotton wool.

to screw into: to connect one thing to another with a circular motion.

to withdraw: to take out.

Mr Peter Cathcart has diabetes. He is admitted to hospital with suspected ketoacidosis. Read this short report from his GP and then answer the questions that follow.

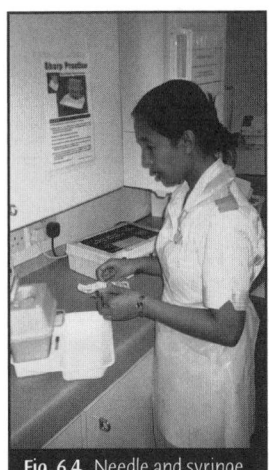

Fig. 6.4 Needle and syringe are assembled.

PATIENT CARE PLAN

Patient:
Peter Cathcart

Age:
46 years

Form of address:
Mr

Occupation:
Bricklayer

Marital status:
Divorced

Medical history:
I have been seeing Mr Cathcart regularly for 10 years. Initially complained of frequent urination (particularly at night), thirst, increased appetite, extreme tiredness and drowsiness which may pose problems when patient is at work on high buildings.
Tests done showed abnormally high levels of glucose. Pancreas clearly not producing adequate insulin for proper metabolism of digested food.
Family history – father diabetic (now deceased).
Diagnosed insulin-dependent diabetes mellitus (IDDM). Though patient requires daily insulin injections, he is forgetful and sometimes neglects to administer these.

Exercise 6g

Say which of the following statements are true:

a The GP says Mr Cathcart is a new patient.
b. Mr Cathcart is single.
c. Mr Cathcart is a skilled worker.
d. The GP complains of a need to frequently use the toilet.
e. The patient's father has diabetes.
f. The patient is often hungry.
g. The patient may have inherited diabetes.
h. The patient's pancreas is functioning normally.
i. The patient is careless about his insulin injections.

Exercise 6h

Say which of the following sentences are grammatically correct.

a. The patient require insulin.
b. The patient is requires insulin.
c. There are a family history of diabetes.
d. The patient is neglectful to give himself injections.
e. The patient neglects to give himself injections.
f. The patient frequently urinates.
g. The patient is frequent urination.
h. The tests are showing high glucose levels.
i. The tests show high glucose levels.
j. The tests have shown high glucose levels.

Exercise 6i   Now complete the following Admission Form for Mr Cathcart by filling in each space with the correct word from the brackets.

PATIENT ADMISSION FORM

Patient's name
Peter Cathcart

Reason for Admission
.... (Excessive, A lot of, Over) ketone production leading to .... (suspected, guessed, assumed) ketoacidosis. This is a potentially life .... (endangered, threatening, risky) condition.

Symptoms
Abdominal .... (in pain, painful, pain), ... (vomiting, vomit, vomited) .... (rapid, quickly, speedy) breathing, ... (extreme, extremely, very) tiredness, ... (drowsy, drowsiness, drowsily).

Action to be taken
Monitor blood sugar levels, ... (give, take, apply) insulin injections.
Dietician .... (to, for, by) discuss diet.
Patient to be shown how to .... (self-monitoring, monitor self, self-monitor) blood glucose (SMBG).
Link SMBG to .... (eat, diet, feed).
Demonstrate to patient how .... (to read, reading, read) SMBG strips.
.... (Emphasise, Stressful, Underlining) importance of monitoring blood sugar levels every morning and keeping record of results to .... (take, brought, fetch) to GP.

Exercise 6j: Further practice

Read this information about a patient and complete the section of the form that follows it:

John Docherty is 19. He is diabetic. This is his fifth admission to hospital. John recently cut his thumb and his GP prescribed a course of oral antibiotics. The next day he was very unwell with pains, nausea, dehydration and polyuria. He was admitted to hospital where he was nursed until his urine was glucose free.

He is an articulate young man with a wide vocabulary. It appears that he knows how to safely inject insulin and is careful to protect himself from infection. He doesn't understand the reasons for this. He passes urine 8 times a day and has regular bowel movements. However, he is getting very little exercise – he works in an office and is driven to work. He is now putting on weight and has started drinking alcohol. Going to the pub is his favourite pastime.

Communication	Eliminating
Safety	Mobility
Eating and drinking	

Answers and comments on the language

Exercise 6a

a. is not true. Her nickname is 'Effie'.

b. is true. A 'live-in partner' is someone you live with but are not formally married to. Sometimes this relationship is called 'common-law husband/wife'.

c. is not true.

d. is not true. Though 'primary' means 'first' or 'most important', the 'primary nurse' is the nurse responsible for admitting the patient.

e. is not true. The term 'uncommunicative' suggests that the patient chooses not to communicate as in the case of Roberta Blackwood (Chapter Five). In Ethel Partridge's case it is best to describe her as: 'unable to communicate.'

f. is true. Note the word 'drowsy' in 'Reason for admission'. Also note that 'to fall' and 'to become' go with 'unconscious'.

g. is not true. Information comes from Robert Greene.

h. is the correct way of saying this. It is interesting that in the case of certain illnesses it is correct to say 'the patient is a…' as in 'the patient is a diabetic' and 'the patient is a schizophrenic'. However, in most cases the patient 'has' or 'suffers from' as in: 'the patient has cancer' or 'the patient is suffering from flu, AIDS', etc.

i. is incorrect.

j. is also a correct way to say it.

Exercise 6b

The patient's breathing is <u>at</u> a rate of 32 per minute and she does not <u>have a cough</u>. Her pulse rate <u>is</u> 128 per minute and her blood pressure is <u>ninety over forty-five</u>. She is <u>of</u> normal body size and has <u>her own teeth</u>. She likes most drinks but <u>has a dislike</u> of milk.

Exercise 6c

When Ethel Partridge was admitted <u>to</u> A&E, she was accompanied <u>by</u> Mr Robert Greene who lives with her. They came <u>by</u> ambulance and Mr Greene reported <u>to</u> staff that his girlfriend had become sleepy, felt generally poorly and then fallen unconscious.

Ethel Partridge is diabetic and will require the supervision <u>of</u> a diabetic nurse specialist in order <u>to</u> learn how <u>to</u> maintain metabolic control <u>in</u> the future. She will need to know <u>of</u> the brain's need <u>for</u> glucose <u>as</u> a source of fuel, the dangers <u>of</u> hypoglycaemia resulting <u>from</u> too much insulin relative <u>to</u> food intake, the relationship <u>between</u> stress and blood sugar levels and methods of testing urine <u>for</u> ketones and blood <u>for</u> sugar.

She needs to know how hyperglycaemia is related <u>to</u> excessive food intake or eating the wrong kinds <u>of</u> food, decreased activity levels <u>in</u> relation <u>to</u> food intake, illness and infections.

Exercise 6d

1   *Question:* Diabetics can't eat sweets, <u>can they</u>?
Answer: Sweets are <u>no worse</u> for diabetics than other people.

2   *Question:* It isn't safe for diabetics to drive, <u>is it</u>?
Answer: Other people are <u>no safer</u> than diabetics.

3   *Question:* <u>Doesn't</u> too much sugar cause diabetes?
Answer: No, it's <u>caused</u> by a combination of things – genes and environment.

4   *Question:* <u>Don't</u> people with diabetes eventually go blind?
Answer: It's possible, but it's <u>less</u> likely if you properly control blood pressure and glucose levels.

5   *Question:* <u>Is it</u> possible to catch diabetes from another person?
Answer: No, we don't know why some people get it, but it <u>isn't</u> contagious.

Exercise 6e

<u>Diabetes</u> was first recorded in <u>ancient</u> Egypt in 1500 BC. The word 'diabetes' <u>is</u> Greek and means 'fountain' referring to the large amounts of <u>urine</u> produced by the disease in its <u>early</u> stages. <u>Diabetic</u> urine smells sweet and its alternative name – 'mellitus' <u>comes</u> from the Latin word for 'honey'. Doctors can often <u>find</u> unsuspected diabetes by <u>finding</u> sugar in routine urine tests. The urine of diabetics attracts ants <u>looking</u> for sugar and early methods of <u>detecting</u> diabetes included <u>tasting</u> the urine for <u>sweetness</u>.

Exercise 6f

1   <u>Assemble</u> a needle and syringe of the correct size, making sure that they both remain aseptic and <u>screw</u> the needle on to the syringe.

2   The needle is <u>inserted</u> through the rubber stopper of the medication bottle.

3   The prescribed dose of the fluid should be <u>withdrawn</u> from the container into the syringe.

4 <u>Turn</u> the bottle and syringe <u>upside down</u> and pull back on the plunger to the required dosage of fluid.

5 <u>Swab</u> the skin at the site chosen for the injection.

6 The syringe needs to be <u>checked</u> for air bubbles.

7 Using the hand you write with, hold the syringe like a pen or pencil and with the other hand <u>pinch</u> about 2 to 3 inches on either side of the skin.

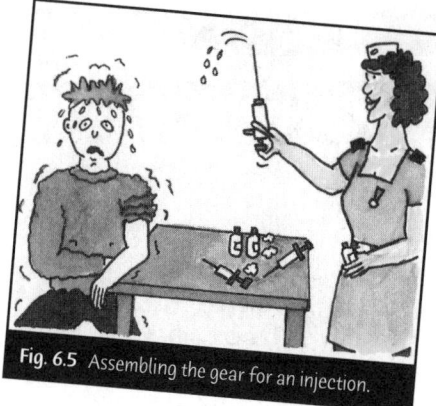

Fig. 6.5 *Assembling the gear for an injection.*

8 About ⅔ of the needle is <u>inserted</u> at a 90° angle.

9 <u>Depress</u> the piston of the syringe.

10 Pull the needle out smoothly and quickly and then <u>dispose</u> of it.

Exercise 6g

a. is not true. Mr Cathcart has been seeing the GP for 10 years.

b. is true. Though Mr Cathcart is officially described as 'divorced', this does mean that he is unmarried – a single man.

c. is true. There are several categories of employment including 'unskilled', 'skilled', 'professional', 'executive', 'self-employed' and 'unemployed'. Bricklayers are trained and usually qualified and therefore categorized as 'skilled'.

d. is not true. When a patient reports symptoms of an illness such as pain this is described as 'complaining of…'. It is not the doctor who is complaining of frequent urination but the patient.

e. is not true. The patient's father is dead. He therefore 'had' diabetes, not 'has' diabetes.

f. is true. 'Increased appetite' suggests feelings of hunger.

g. is true. The patient's father was diabetic. People 'inherit' characteristics from parents, etc.

h. is not true.

i. is true. This is one of several ways of saying 'neglects (to do something)'.

Exercise 6h

The following sentences are grammatically correct:

e.

f.

h.

i.

j.

Exercise 6i

PATIENT CARE PLAN

Patients Name
Peter Cathcart

Reason for admission
<u>Excessive</u> ketone production leading to <u>suspected</u> ketoacidosis. This is a potentially life-<u>threatening</u> condition.

Symptoms
Abdominal <u>pain</u>, <u>vomiting</u>, <u>rapid</u> breathing, <u>extreme</u> tiredness, <u>drowsiness</u>.

Action to be taken
Monitor blood sugar levels, <u>give</u> insulin injections.
Dietician <u>to</u> discuss diet.
Patient to be shown how to <u>self-monitor</u> blood glucose (SMBG).
Link SMBG to <u>diet</u>.
Demonstrate to patient how <u>to read</u> SMBG strips.
<u>Emphasise</u> importance of monitoring blood sugar levels every morning and keeping record of results to <u>take</u> to GP.

Exercise 6j: Further practice

Communication
Articulate. Good vocab.

Safety
Knows how to inject insulin & guard against infection
Does not know *why*.

Eating and drinking
Difficulty keeping to modified diet. Drinks alcohol. Putting on weight.

Eliminating
Urine 8 × daily.

Mobility
Very little exercise. Does not walk to work, sedentary job.
Spends spare time drinking in pub.

Chapter Seven

Paul Marston – head injury

Read the following case notes on a patient who has had an accident:

The patient is a ten-year-old boy called Paul Marston. The following information comes from him, his father and the ambulance crew.

VOCABULARY

crew: paramedics operating an ambulance.

helmet: head protection.

handlebars: part of a bicycle used for steering.

to complain of: to report a pain or illness.

nausea: a sense of feeling sick.

pre-school: before starting school.

alert: aware of everything that's going on.

tender(ness): hurts when you touch it.

gait: walking movement.

to trim: (to make) tidy.

brisk: sharp, immediately responsive.

ragged: not tidy.

transverse: from one side to the other.

laceration: cut.

History

On his way to school this morning, the patient was cycling down hill when he lost control of his bicycle. The front wheel hit the kerb and he flew over the handlebars. His head and right shoulder hit the pavement (he was not wearing a helmet) and he was unconscious for about 2 minutes.

When the ambulance arrived, he was confused but he was sitting up talking. He walked into the ambulance and vomited once on the way to the hospital. The patient's next memory is of being in the ambulance (i.e. PTA was approx. 10–15 minutes). On admission he complained of having a headache all over. After vomiting, there was no nausea and he did not complain of pain anywhere else.

PMH

The patient takes no medications and does not suffer from any allergies. He had a pre-school tetanus booster 4 years ago.

Observations and examination

The examination shows that he is a fit child, fully alert and orientated. He has a 5-cm ragged, transverse laceration across the left frontal region just below the hairline.

He has full movement in both eyes. Both eyes are strong and he has brisk reflexes. There is no tenderness in his neck, no sign of trauma to his left shoulder and no evidence of any other injury. Spine and chest are OK and he has no pain in his ribs. The patient's abdomen is soft, pelvis is OK, legs are OK and he walks with a normal gait.

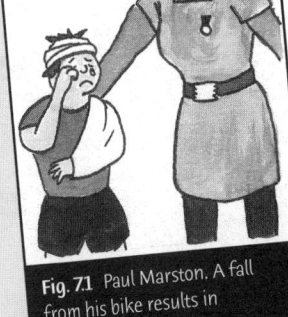

Fig. 7.1 Paul Marston. A fall from his bike results in admission to A & E.

Diagnosis

The patient has suffered a minor head injury with a possible PTA of 15 minutes with laceration.

Treatment

The wound is cleaned, the edges of the wound are trimmed and the patient's head receives 6 Ethilon sutures. His father is advised to give paracetamol and to see Practice Nurse for the sutures to be taken out.

Exercise 7a   **Choose the correct answer for each of the following questions:**

1   On an assessment form there might be a section called 'Prefers to be addressed as'. This is asking about:
a. the patient's surname.
b. the patient's home.
c. the patient's nickname.

2   On an assessment form, 'Family's Understanding of Admission' asks the question:
a. does the family understand why the patient is being admitted?
b. what does the family believe is the reason for admitting the patient?
c. is the family in favour of admitting the patient?

3   On an assessment form the 'nurse's initial impression' is:
a. the nurse's main impression of the patient.
b. the nurse's opinion about the admission.
c. the nurse's first thoughts about the patient.

4   According to the text, Paul Marston:
a. fell over his bicycle.
b. fell on his bicycle.
c. fell off his bicycle.

5   When the ambulance came, the patient:
a. was walking.
b. was able to walk.
c. refused to walk.

6   On admission, the patient:
a. had head pains.
b. made a complaint about his head.
c. had pains all over.

7   The laceration on the patient's head is:
a. vertical.
b. horizontal.
c. diagonal.

Exercise 7b   Now complete Paul Marston's Patient Assessment Form by making a choice from a, b or c for each entry on the form. Sometimes when more than one choice is possible, you must choose the best.

PATIENT ASSESSMENT RECORD

Patient's name: Paul Marston

Prefers to be addressed as: Paul

Reason for admission
a. Involved in road accident.
b. Lacerated forehead, headache + PTA 2 min.
c. Minor head injury, unconscious approx. 2 min.

Family's understanding of admission: injured in accident

Patient's understanding of admission:
a. fell off bike, cut on head.
b. confused about accident.
c. feeling sick.

Medical diagnosis:
a. lacerated head with PTA of poss. 15 min.
b. Injured head. Poss. PTA 15 min.
c. Poss. injury to head with 15-min PTA.

Nurse's initial impression (physical and social):
a. patient active, alert, no apparent problems besides injury.
b. patient disorientated but not traumatised.
c. patient active and alert, no signs of any kind of injury.

Exercise 7c

This is a list of some of the possible consequences of a blow to the head. Use the information in the list to complete the text that follows the list. As you insert things from the list, you will have to make changes to the words.

Effects of head injuries

Physical
decrease of motor speed
poor co-ordination

Cognitive
losing memory
speech slurring
losing sense of time and space

Behavioural
irritability
verbal and physical aggressiveness

The paramedics at the scene of the accident noted that the patient, Paul Marston (age 10 years) had been unconscious for two minutes. When he regained consciousness, his .... (meaning: speed of physical movement) had .... and for a time he was .... (meaning: couldn't accurately touch his nose with his finger).

When the paramedics asked him questions there were signs of .... (meaning: couldn't remember) and the patient's speech was .... (meaning: not clear). For a short time, the patient .... (meaning: unaware of where he was and what time it was).

These effects were temporary and if there are any behavioural changes such as becoming .... (meaning: spoken or physical violence) and .... (meaning: easily gets angry) then these will appear over the next few days to family members and be reported to the family doctor.

Exercise 7d

Paul Marston's treatment includes sutures which will be removed later by the Practice Nurse. Fill in the gaps in the following instructions for removing sutures.

Remove .... (some, the, a) dressing, expose the wound and clean .... (them, it, they) with antiseptic solution and a fresh swab. Hold the knot of the first suture with forceps which .... (was, had been, have been) sterilised. .... (Undo, Start, Open) the stitch cutter and slide the blade under the suture, close .... (to, by, at) where it meets ...... (a, the, some) skin. Cut the suture and then .... (softly, quietly, gently) pull it out with .... (the, a, some) forceps. Repeat this operation ...... (on, in, by) every other suture and when you .... (are removing, have removed, remove) half of the sutures, if the wound .... (remain, remaining, remains) intact, take out the rest.

Exercise 7e

Which of these things are 'made' and which are 'done'? Which ones can be either made or done? Use some version of 'make' or 'do' to complete each of the sentences:

a. An examination. A careful examination was .... of the wound.
b. A wound. The boy's fall .... a nasty wound in his forehead.
c. A hole. The doctor will .... two tiny holes. Here and here.
d. A test. The nurse will .... a test for reflexes.
e. A measurement. We have .... a measurement of blood alcohol.
f. A recovery. We expect the patient .... a full recovery.
g. An improvement. Though still poorly he has .... a dramatic improvement.
h. A diagnosis. When we've got the test results back we can perhaps .... a diagnosis.
i. Surgery. We will have to .... minor surgery on the patient's head.
j. An assessment. After .... an assessment of the situation, we will be clearer about what to do next.

Describing shapes and positions

Paul Marston has 'a 5-cm ragged, transverse laceration across the left frontal region just below the hairline.' (It is 5 cm long, untidy, horizontal and on his left forehead). For some general practice in describing shapes, sizes and positions look at this vocabulary and follow the instructions after it:

Exercise 7f

Instructions:

Draw a horizontal rectangle approximately 6 cm by 4 cm.

On the upper side of the rectangle, draw a triangle with sides of equal length so that one side of the triangle is the length of the rectangle.

At the apex of the triangle, draw a circle with a radius of 2 cm so that the apex of the triangle touches the centre of the circle.

Check your finished drawing with the one in the 'Answers' section.

VOCABULARY

Triangle (adjective: triangular)

Circle (adjective: circular) and 4 sectors

Horizontal line

Vertical line

Diagonal line

Rectangle (adjective: rectangular)

Right angle (adjective: right angled)

Exercise 7g

Put single words into the spaces in these sentences:

a. The surgeon made a .... incision with the scalpel. (meaning: a cut with three sides)
b. Hold the dropper .... (meaning: straight up)
c. Ensure the patient sleeps as .... as possible. (meaning: flat)
d. Set the equipment at .... to the floor. (meaning: at 90°)
e. Use the catheter with the .... end. (meaning: round)
f. The .... bowl can be used for disposables. (meaning: not square but with four sides)
g. If the blue .... changes colour, the test is positive. (meaning: part of a circle)

Describing mathematical formulae

Exercise 7h

Here is a typical calculation which has to be made by nurses in their work:

A patient is prescribed 45 mg of loxapine which has to be given by injection. However, 50 mg of loxapine is in 1 ml of liquid. The question is, how many ml of the liquid should be administered to the patient to make up the correct dose?

You get the answer by doing the following sum: 45 mg (the required dose) ÷ 50 mg (the stocked dose) = 0.9 (ml). When written in English this sum is: 'forty-five divided by fifty equals nought point nine millilitres.'

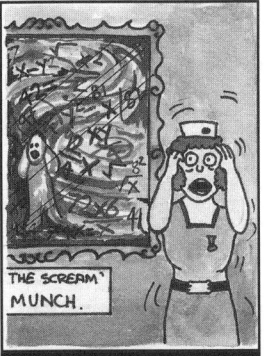

Fig. 7.2 There is no escape from mathematics.

VOCABULARY

÷: divide, into, e.g. 5 ÷ 2 is written: 'five divided by two' or 'two into five'

×: multiply, times, e.g. 5 × 2 is written: 'five multiplied by two' or 'five times two' or 'five by two'.

+: add, plus, e.g. 5 + 2 is written 'five add two' or 'five plus two'.

−: minus, subtract, take away, e.g. 5 − 2 is written 'five minus two' or 'five subtract two' or 'five take away two.'

=: equals, e.g. 5 + 2 = 7 is written 'five plus two equals seven' or 'five plus two is equal to seven', etc.

Put the following sums into words:

a. $7 + 5 \times 3 = 36$

b. $453 \div 3 = 151$

c. $6700 + 95 - 333 \times 2 = 12\ 724$

d. $x^2 \times \sqrt{y^3} = 5$

e. the area of a circle is $\pi \times radius^2$

Exercise 7i

Sandra Dawkins is three years old. Her GP phones the hospital to prepare for an admission and her parents accompany her in an ambulance. Sandra has been weepy for the past two days and sometimes crying inconsolably. She has been running a temperature of around 104° F (40° C.) She has a nasty-looking rash on her neck and shoulders. She has a lot of mucus in her nose and throat and has difficulty breathing. Her parents report no diarrhoea though she vomited once an hour before seeing the doctor.

A diagnosis is required and in the meantime the doctor recommends that she should be given as much fluid as possible to drink in order to avoid dehydration as a result of her fever (though no drinks containing caffeine). Also that she be dressed lightly, with light bedclothes and that she be given a lukewarm sponge bath.

From the above information, say which of the following statements are true:

a. The child has been running around and made herself hot.
b. She grows quieter when she is comforted.
c. Nothing seems to stop her from crying.
d. It is OK for her to drink Coca Cola if she will take it.
e. She should be immersed in warm water.

Exercise 7j

Now choose the correct entries to make on the following clinical form from the choices of a, b and c.

PATIENT ADMISSION FORM	**Initial impression**
	a. Rash, fever, parents report no vomiting.
Patient	b. Rash, high temp., parents report little vomiting.
Sandra Dawkins	c. Rash, temp., vomited.

Base-line functions	**Possible problems**
a. Temp: 104°c.	a. Dehydration.
b. Temp: 40°f.	b. Dehydrated.
c. Temp:104°f.	c. Rehydration.

Reason for admission	**Nursing instructions**
a. High temp., diarrhoea, vomiting.	a. Encourage to drink ql. Wash at blood temp. No heavy blankets.
b. Fever, finds breathing difficult.	b. Lower temp. and rehydrate.
c. Crying a lot, dehydrated.	c. Bathe in cool water, provide drinks ql, to wear light-coloured clothing.

Answers and comments on the language

Exercise 7a

1   c. However, sometimes a 'nickname' is not a name you like but one given to you by other people. 'Address' here refers to a name. You 'address' someone by name. People have a 'title' (also called 'form of address') which can be 'Mister', 'Doctor', 'Professor', etc. (see Chapter Five, Exercise 5b).

2   b. An 'understanding of' something here refers not to whether you understand it but <u>what</u> you understand or <u>how much</u> you understand.

3   c. 'Initial' means 'first'. Your 'initials' are the first letters of your name.

4   c. If the patient had fallen 'over' or fallen 'on' his bike he would not have been riding it.

5   b.

6   a. A 'pain in the head' can become a 'head pain', a 'pain in the stomach' can become 'stomach pain', etc. To 'complain of pain' is to say that you are in pain. This is different from 'to make a complaint' (option **b**) which suggests that the patient's head has done something wrong and he is informing a higher authority.

7   b.

Exercise 7b

Reason for admission

c. is the best choice. To be 'involved' in a road accident (option **a**) is not in itself a reason for admission. Option **b** is inaccurate. PTA was 10–15 minutes.

Patient's understanding of admission

a. is the best choice. Option **b** is not 'an understanding of admission' and option **c** is not a reason for admission.

Medical diagnosis

a. Note the position of 'poss.' (possible). Option **b** says that the PTA is possible – which it isn't – it is definite. Option **c** says the patient has a possible injury to the head whereas in fact the injury is definite.

Nurse's initial impression

a. By the time the patient arrives at the hospital he is no longer disorientated (option **b**). Option **c** is wrong.

Exercise 7c

The paramedics at the scene of the accident noted that the patient, Paul Marston (age 10 years) had been unconscious for two minutes. When he regained consciousness his <u>motor speed</u> had <u>decreased</u> and for a time he was <u>poorly co-ordinated</u>.

When the paramedics asked him questions there were signs of <u>loss of memory</u> and the patient's speech was <u>slurred</u>. For a short time, the patient <u>lost his sense of time and space</u>.

These effects were temporary and if there are any behavioural changes such as becoming <u>verbally and physically aggressive</u> and <u>irritable</u>, then these will appear over the next few days to family members and be reported to the family doctor.

Exercise 7d

Remove <u>the</u> dressing, expose the wound and clean <u>it</u> with antiseptic solution and a fresh swab. Hold the knot of the first suture with forceps which <u>have been</u> sterilised. <u>Open</u> the stitch cutter and slide the blade under the suture, close <u>to</u> where it meets <u>the</u> skin. Cut the suture and then <u>gently</u> pull it out with <u>the</u> forceps. Repeat this operation <u>on</u> every other suture and when you <u>have removed</u> half of the sutures, if the wound <u>remains</u> intact, take out the rest.

Exercise 7e

a. Do or make an examination. A careful examination was <u>made/done</u> of the wound.
b. Make a wound. The boy's fall <u>made</u> a nasty wound in his forehead.
c. Make a hole. The doctor will <u>make</u> two tiny holes. Here and here.
d. Do a test. The nurse will <u>do</u> a test for reflexes.
e. Make or do a measurement. We have <u>made/done</u> a measurement for blood alcohol level.
f. Make a recovery. We expect the patient <u>to make</u> a full recovery.
g. Make an improvement. Though still poorly he has <u>made</u> a dramatic improvement.
h. Make or do a diagnosis. When we've got the test results back we can perhaps <u>make/do</u> a diagnosis.
i. Do surgery. We will have to <u>do</u> minor surgery on the patient's head.
j. Make or do an assessment. After <u>making/doing</u> an assessment of the situation we will be clearer about what to do next.

Exercise 7f

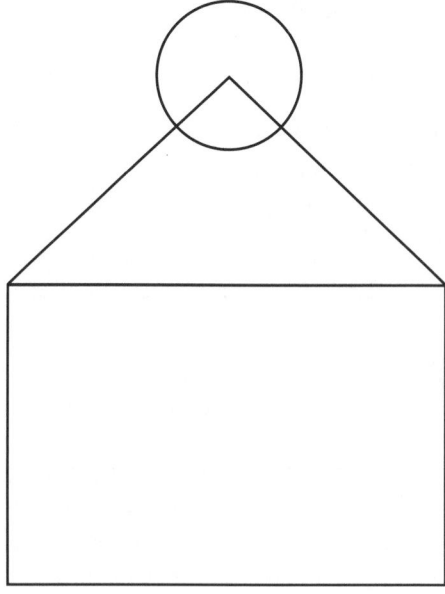

Exercise 7g

a. The surgeon made a <u>triangular</u> incision with the scalpel.
b. Hold the dropper <u>vertically</u>.
c. Ensure the patient sleeps as <u>horizontally</u> as possible.
d. Set the equipment at <u>right angles</u> to the floor.
e. Use the catheter with the <u>circular</u> end.
f. The <u>rectangular</u> bowl can be used for disposables.
g. If the blue <u>sector</u> changes colour, the test is positive.

Exercise 7h

a. Seven plus five multiplied by three equals thirty-six. Or: Seven add five times three is equal to thirty-six.
b. Four hundred and fifty-three divided by three is equal to one hundred and fifty-one. Or: Three into four hundred and fifty-three equals one hundred and fifty-one.
c. Six thousand seven hundred add ninety-five take away three hundred and thirty-three, times two equals twelve thousand seven hundred and twenty-four.
d. x squared times/multiplied by/the square root of y cubed/the cube of y equals five.
e. The area of a circle is pi times the radius squared. Or: The area of a circle equals pi multiplied by the square of the radius.

Exercise 7i

a. is not true. The text says she is 'running a temperature'. This means she has a high temperature.
b. is not true. The text says she is 'inconsolable'. This means nothing will comfort her and stop her from crying.
c. is true. (see above – **b**)
d. is not true. Coca Cola is a caffeinated drink.
e. is not true. A 'sponge bath' is an all over wash using a sponge or flannel.

Exercise 7j

Patient	
Sandra Dawkins	
Base-line functions	
c. Temp: 104°f	
Reason for admission	
b. Fever, finds breathing difficult.	
Initial impression	
c. Rash, temp, vomited.	
Possible problems	
a. Dehydration	
Nursing instructions	
a. Encourage to drink ql. Wash at blood temp. No heavy blankets.	

Chapter Eight

Accidents and emergencies

On the next page there is a Road Traffic Accident (RTA) Information Sheet. Read it carefully, then do Exercises 8a and 8b.

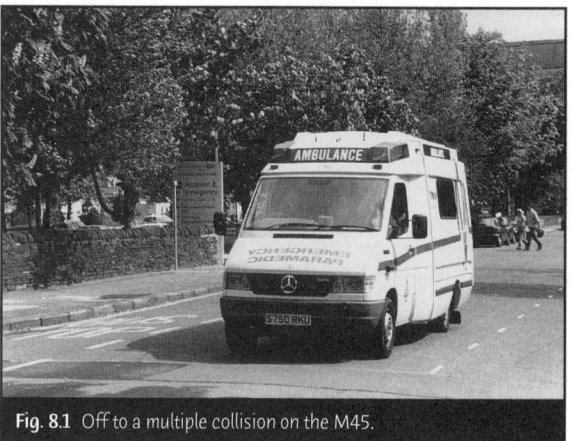

Fig. 8.1 Off to a multiple collision on the M45.

Exercise 8a

From the details given on the form above, say which of the following statements are true:

a. The patient had been in the back of the car.

b. The patient got out of the car himself.

c. The patient was thrown out of the car during the crash.

d. The patient's car turned over.

e. The patient has been exposed to dangerous chemicals.

Exercise 8b

Now read this report of the accident and fill in the gaps with the correct choice of word(s) from the brackets:

At 10.30 p.m. Albert Thomas was .... (admit, be admitted, admitted) to the A&E Department. The patient .... (has been, were, had been) in a road accident. He was unconscious .... (on, in, at) arrival suffering multiple .... (injury, injured, injuries) to head, neck and legs.

RTA Information (circle the appropriate response)

Patient's name
Albert Thomas

How was the patient travelling?
Lorry
Bus
Van
(Car)
Motorcycle
Bicycle
Pedestrian

What was the patient doing at the time of the RTA?
Driver
(FS passenger)
Rear Right passenger
Rear Left Passenger
Motorcycle rider
Pillion passenger

What was the direction of impact? (show with arrows)

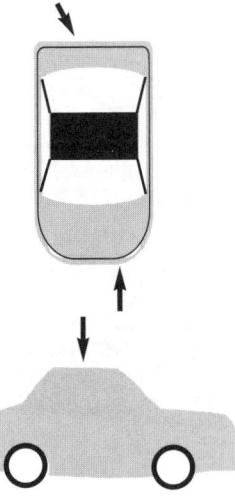

What damage was done to the vehicle?
(Front)
RS
LS
(Rear)
(Roof)
Bottom

What intrusion was there?
(Roof)
Steering column
Floor
Wheel arch
Door(s)

What happened to the patient at the time of the RTA?
Patient was:
Ejected
Run over
Hit by other vehicle
Immersed
Burnt
Injured by chemicals
(Trapped)

What part of the vehicle did the patient come in contact with?
Steering wheel
Dashboard
Screen
Crash helmet
Other

If on bicycle/motorcycle, was patient wearing crash-helmet?
Yes
No

The patient .... (have been, used to be, had been) a front seat passenger in a car which was in a multiple collision on the M45 .... (involving, involved, to involved) a lorry and four cars. Apart from the patient and the driver, there were .... (none, not, no) other people in their vehicle. The driver of one of the other cars .... (were, be, was) injured and taken to hospital but the lorry driver was unhurt.

The car the patient had been .... (travelling, travel, travelled) in struck the rear of the lorry and was then hit from .... (back, rear, behind) by a second car. The patient's car turned .... (under, into, over) and the roof of his vehicle was forced inwards and probably caused some of the injuries to his head and neck. The patient had been .... (trap, traps, trapped) in the vehicle for approximately ten minutes before he was .... (release, released, to be released) by the emergency services that arrived on the scene.

Exercise 8c

Now read this report about another car accident and with the information complete the RTA form that follows. Compare your form with the completed one in the Answers section.

RTA REPORT

This patient is an elderly woman, Mrs Dorothy Brown. She was admitted to A&E at 4.45 p.m. She had been in a road accident approximately forty minutes earlier. When she was admitted to hospital, Mrs Brown was fully conscious and able to talk coherently. However, she was suffering from shock and she was vague about what had happened. A policeman gave staff a description of what he knew about the accident.

Mrs Brown had been driving along Riverside Road when she hit a stationary tanker carrying chlorine parked at the side of the road on a blind bend. The front of her car was seriously damaged, the steering wheel was pushed forward by the impact and came into contact with the lower part of Mrs Brown's face and chest. Chemicals did escape from the tanker but it was not clear on admission if Mrs Brown had come into contact with them.

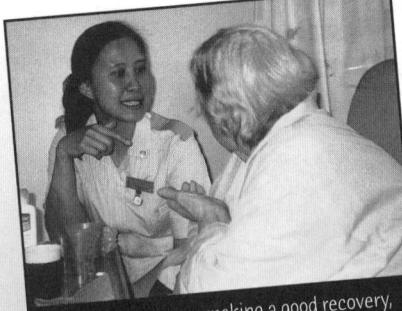

Fig. 8.2 Mrs Brown, making a good recovery, chats to a nurse.

RTA Information (circle the appropriate response)

Patient's name

How was the patient travelling?
Lorry
Bus
Van
Car
Motorcycle
Bicycle
Pedestrian

What was the patient doing at the time of the RTA?
Driver
FS passenger
Rear Right passenger
Rear Left Passenger
Motorcycle rider
Pillion passenger

What was the direction of impact? (show with arrows)

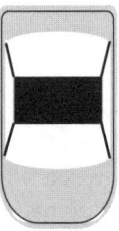

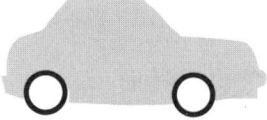

What damage was done to the vehicle?
Front
RS
LS
Rear
Roof
Bottom

What intrusion was there?
Roof
Steering column
Floor
Wheel arch
Door(s)

What happened to the patient at the time of the RTA?
Patient was:
Ejected
Run over
Hit by other vehicle
Immersed
Burnt
Injured by chemicals
Trapped

What part of the vehicle did the patient come in contact with?
Steering wheel
Dashboard
Screen
Crash helmet
Other

If on bicycle/motorcycle, was patient wearing crash-helmet?
Yes
No

Exercise 8d   First look at the words in the vocabulary list. Then put the correct forms of the words into the gaps in the text which follows (the first one is done for you):

VOCABULARY

to dislocate: displace bones. To move (bones) out of their proper position.

neighbouring: next to.

crutch: device for helping people walk with leg injuries.

to swell: to increase in size.

palm: flat part of an open hand.

to strap: to fix firmly into place using a strip of material of some kind.

a pad: a wad to give protection from bumps and knocks.

stiff: does not move naturally and easily.

to be untreated: to be neglected and not given medical treatment when it is needed.

sling: the cloth that goes around the patient's neck and holds their arm steady.

collar: neck support.

to stub: to knock your toe against something.

to elevate: raise/lift up.

digit: finger or toe.

temder: hurts when touched.

Advice for the nursing care of injured patients

Fractures and <u>dislocations</u> (dislocate) of toes are often caused by a .... (stub) toe. Treat by .... (strap) the injured toe to a neighbouring digit for support. Use gauze .... (pad) and watch out for any .... (swell).

Treat metatarsal fractures by .... (elevate) the foot and ensure that the foot is NWB. Ensure the patient rests and uses two .... (crutch) for essential walking. Watch out for .... (swell) and any neurovascular damage.

Wrist injuries are often caused by falls onto .... (palm) of the hand. Fractures often do not show up on the first X-ray. If there is .... (local) .... (tender) treat as if it were a fracture. If the injury is left .... (untreat) there is a risk of osteoarthritis. Falls in the elderly often cause upper-arm fractures. Use a sling or a collar but remember that it is important to keep mobility to prevent permanent .... (stiff).

Exercise 8e   The following is advice given to medical staff about how to speak to patients brought in for an emergency ECG assessment of chest pain. Choose from a, b and c which has the closest meaning to the underlined part of each sentence:

1   In an emergency situation, chest pain is a very frightening experience and <u>fear can make the condition worse</u>.
   a. patients will get scared if the chest pain gets worse.
   b. the fear that is created by pain may increase the pain.
   c. the greater the pain, the greater the fear.

2   Before performing an ECG, <u>the nurse should explain in a language the patient can understand</u> exactly what is to be done and why.
   a. The nurse should not use jargon.
   b. The nurse should speak her mind.
   c. The nurse should not speak in her own language.

3 You might have to tell a patient that: <u>the ECG machine records heart rhythm and assists with an assessment of the origins of pain.</u>

   a. 'The ECG machine may cause you a little pain.'
   b. 'The ECG will give us information about why you're in pain.'
   c. 'The recording will tell us whether or not you are in pain.'

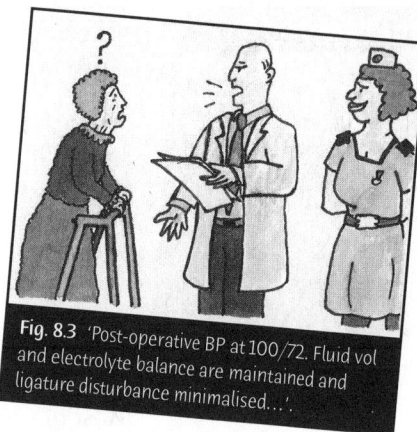

Fig. 8.3 'Post-operative BP at 100/72. Fluid vol and electrolyte balance are maintained and ligature disturbance minimalised...'.

4 Unfortunately sometimes <u>a doctor will tell the patient nothing.</u>

   a. Some doctors don't say nothing to patients.
   b. No doctors will give information to patients.
   c. Some doctors don't tell their patients anything.

5 Speak in Plain English. If, for example, you tell a patient that you are going <u>to make an electrocardiographic recording of their heart</u>, say.

   a. 'Your heart will be recorded by an ECG.'
   b. 'The ECG is a tracing of your heart.'
   c. 'This will show us what your heart is doing.'

Exercise 8f

Read the following clinical instructions for routine ear-syringing. You will see that 'passive' sentences are used. Change the passive sentences into active ones, e.g. 'the external canal is examined' becomes: 'examine the external canal.'

1 Using the auriscope, the external canal and eardrum are examined.

....

2 The syringe is primed with the solution.

....

3 Protective covering is placed over the patient's shoulder.

....

4 The pinna of the ear is gently pulled in an upwards and backwards direction to straighten out the canal.

....

5 The fluid is introduced through the syringe.

....

6 After the canal has been examined again to assess the result of the syringing, the canal is carefully dried.

....

Exercise 8g

Where there is a number in the following article, write it out in words.

Beware of the tea cosy

3 000 000 .... people are injured in their homes in the UK every year and 4000 .... of them die. The UK Government has compiled information based on hospital admissions about domestic accidents and a government report is available.

The report says that in 1999 there were 10 773 .... cases of people treated for accidents caused by socks and tights, 5945 .... accidents caused by trousers and 1317 .... by beanbags. Most of these were falls caused by getting stuck in rushed attempts to get dressed in untidy bedrooms.

Vegetables caused 13 132 .... accidents in 1999. The report is not clear about how a vegetable can cause an accident but it is probably because when casualty patients are asked 'what happened?' they say something like, 'it was the mushrooms' and this gets written down as a 'cause'.

1771 .... accidents were caused by leaves, 787 .... by loofahs and sponges and 37 .... by tea-cosies, which is an increase from 20 .... in the previous year. Most of the tea-cosy injuries were scalds caused by picking up a tea-pot by its cosy rather than its handle or tripping up on tea-cosies on slippery kitchen floors.

False teeth caused 933 .... accidents, toilet-roll holders 329 ...., dustpans 146 .... and bread-bins 91 .... A total of 16 662 .... people had to go to hospital after accidents with a sofa and 5615

....
after an accident with a wellington boot.

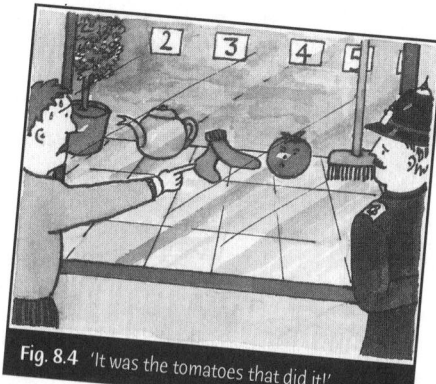

Fig. 8.4 'It was the tomatoes that did it!'

Report on Mrs Nolan

Mrs Nolan is an elderly woman who is brought in to Accident and Emergency after a fall at home in which she badly bruised and cut her face and arms. This report follows soon after her. It comes from a District Nurse who regularly visits Mrs Nolan at home.

REPORT

Patient: Mrs Margaret Nolan

Mrs Nolan is 77 years old. She lives with her husband.

Mrs Nolan had a small stroke 13 months ago and now needs some assistance with ADLs. No full assessment has been made by her GP about her cognitive state. There is a note from her GP describing her as 'somewhat disoriented'. Her GP has prescribed antidepressants.

Mr Nolan expresses concern about his wife. He has described her as 'agitated, confused, and depressed'.

Mr Nolan is 88. He is frail and suffers from hearing difficulties. He says he is doing 'just fine' at home, though his son nags him to get help with Mrs Nolan.

Mr Nolan reports that his wife is up and down all night long and wanders through the house in the dark.

Mrs Nolan attends Eastchester Adult Day Care Centre. Staff there report that she seldom converses and that she gets up from activities and wanders around the building trying doors and talks about going for a walk. At other times she is very lethargic. She has difficulty following directions and there is occasional urinary incontinence.

As yet, no specific psychiatric diagnosis has been provided.

Exercise 8h   **Answer the following questions by choosing the best answer from a, b and c.**

1   How often has a District Nurse visited Mrs Nolan at home?
a. Occasionally.
b. On occasion.
c. At intervals.

2   How much assistance with ADLs does Mrs Nolan need?
a. A little.
b. A lot.
c. None.

3   What does 'somewhat disoriented' mean?
a. Extremely disoriented.
b. Sometimes disoriented.
c. A bit disoriented.

4   What does Mr Nolan mean by 'just fine'?
a. There are no problems.
b. I am only just managing.
c. I won't be able to handle things much longer.

5 Why does his son nag him?
a. He thinks there is no need for help.
b. He thinks his father needs help.
c. He thinks his mother should have help.

6 Mrs Nolan 'seldom converses' at the Day Centre. What does this mean?
a. She likes a chat.
b. She is withdrawn.
c. She is very serious.

7 What does 'wandering' through the house suggest?
a. Mrs Nolan is aimless.
b. Mrs Nolan is clumsy.
c. She always follows the same route.

8 What do they mean when the Day Care staff say that Mrs Nolan is 'at other times lethargic'?
a. Sometimes she is lazy.
b. She will occasionally sit blankly.
c. She is in turn very active then very passive.

9 Which alternative way of saying 'occasional urinary incontinence' is grammatically correct?
a. Sometimes incontinent of urine.
b. Occasionally incontinence of urine.
c. Sometimes incontinent urine.

10 What does the District Nurse's comment 'no specific diagnosis has been provided' suggest?
a. No diagnosis fits Mrs Nolan's case.
b. The District Nurse has not yet made a diagnosis.
c. The District Nurse is waiting for someone to make a diagnosis.

Exercise 8i

The report on Mrs Nolan is summarised here. Fill in the gaps in the summary with a word from each of the brackets.

Mrs Nolan is an .... (old age, age old, elderly) woman and having suffered .... (the, a, this) stroke now needs assistance in her .... (day, daily, day-by-day) life. Her husband, who is old and frail, is perhaps .... (finding, finds, find) it difficult .... (to cope, cope, be coping) at home. Mrs Nolan is often .... (disturbance, disturbing, disturbed) and .... (distress, distressing, distressed) and the Day Care staff who know her say that she is either .... (hyperactive, hyperactivity, hyperactively) or sits .... (lethargically, lethargic, lethargy). So far she has not .... (be assessed, being assessed, been assessed) by a psychiatrist.

Exercise 8i: Further practice

Use information from these notes to complete the form that follows.

The patient is a two-year-old girl – Jacqueline Johnson (her parents call her 'Jackie'). She was admitted with superficial burns to her left arm, chest and face. It appears that she pulled down a saucepan of very hot water from the cooker and scalded herself. On admission her temperature was recorded as 38.2°C.

Her mother brought her in. She told staff that Jackie has started to speak single words. She is a 'good eater' who eats and drinks almost anything, though prefers fruit juice to milk and likes sweets a lot. She is still in nappies and has bowel movements usually twice a day. She calls both faeces and urine 'wee wee'. When a nurse removed her nappy, her stools were slightly discoloured and strong-smelling. Her breathing is at a rate of 35/min and pulse rate 128/min.

Jacqueline is an active child though her mother says she cries a lot. Her favourite toy is a clown called 'Ham'. She loves it when people read to her.

PATIENT ADMISSION FORM		
Patient's name		
Preferred form of address		
Reason for admission		
Source of information		
Base-line functions	Temp. Respiration	Circulation
Communication		
Elimination		
Work and play		
Eating and drinking		

Answers and comments on the language

Exercise 8a

a. is not true. The patient was a front seat passenger (FS).

b. is not true. The patient was trapped in the car.

c. is not true.

d. is true. On the basis of the evidence of the damage to the vehicle, you can be fairly sure that the car turned over. Not only are the front and back damaged, but also the roof which 'intruded' and probably injured the patient.

e. is not true. There is no evidence of this on the RTA Form.

Exercise 8b

At 10.30 p.m. Albert Thomas was <u>admitted</u> to the A&E Department. The patient <u>had been</u> in a road accident. He was unconscious <u>on</u> arrival suffering multiple <u>injuries</u> to head, neck and legs.

The patient <u>had been</u> a front seat passenger in a car which was in a multiple collision on the M45 <u>involving</u> a lorry and four cars. Apart from the patient and the driver, there were <u>no</u> other people in their vehicle. The driver of one of the other cars <u>was</u> injured and taken to hospital but the lorry driver was unhurt.

The car the patient had been <u>travelling</u> in struck the rear of the lorry and was then hit from <u>behind</u> by a second car. The patient's car turned <u>over</u> and the roof of his vehicle was forced inwards and probably caused some of the injuries to his head and neck. The patient had been <u>trapped</u> in the vehicle for approximately ten minutes before he was <u>released</u> by the emergency services that arrived on the scene.

Exercise 8c

RTA Information (CIRCLE THE APPROPRIATE RESPONSE)

Patient's name
Mrs Dorothy Brown

How was the patient travelling?
Lorry
Bus
Van
(Car)
Motorcycle
Bicycle
Pedestrian

What was the patient doing at the time of the RTA?
(Driver)
FS passenger
Rear Right passenger
Rear Left Passenger
Motorcycle rider
Pillion passenger

What was the direction of impact? (show with arrows)

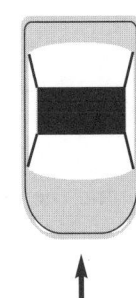
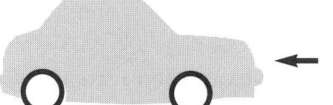

What damage was done to the vehicle?
(Front)
RS
LS
Rear
Roof
Bottom

What intrusion was there?
Roof
(Steering column)
Floor
Wheel arch
Door(s)

What happened to the patient at the time of the RTA?
Patient was:
Ejected
Run over
Hit by other vehicle
Immersed
Burnt
(Injured by chemicals?)**?**
Trapped

What part of the vehicle did the patient come in contact with?
(Steering wheel)
Dashboard
Screen
Crash helmet
Other

If on bicycle/motorcycle was patient wearing crash-helmet?
Yes   N/A
No

Exercise 8d

Fractures and <u>dislocations</u> of toes are often caused by a <u>stubbed</u> toe. Treat by <u>strapping</u> the injured toe to a neighbouring digit for support. Use gauze <u>padding</u> and watch out for any <u>swelling</u>.

Treat metatarsal fractures by <u>elevating</u> the foot and ensure that the foot is NWB. Ensure the patient rests and uses two <u>crutches</u> for essential walking. Watch out for <u>swelling</u> and any neurovascular damage.

Wrist injuries are often caused by falls onto <u>the palm</u> of the hand. Fractures often do not show up on the first X-ray. If there is <u>localised/local tenderness</u> treat as if it were a fracture. If the injury is left <u>untreated</u> there is a risk of osteoarthritis. Falls in the elderly often cause upper-arm fractures. Use a sling or a collar but remember that it is important to keep mobility to prevent permanent <u>stiffness</u>.

Exercise 8e

1. b. The word 'scared' in option **a** means the same as 'to be afraid of'. You can say: 'the patient is scared of injections' and this is the same as 'the patient is afraid of injections' or 'the patient fears injections'.

2. a. The word 'language' here refers to style of language and methods of explaining things. 'Jargon' is words and expressions which are specific to jobs and areas of study so nursing has its own jargon which is not understood by people who are not nurses. 'To speak your mind' (option **b**) is to tell someone what you think. Often the person 'speaking their mind' is angry.

3. b. Option **c** is not right because the sentence questions whether or not there is pain. The patient, of course, knows there is pain.

4. c. Note that 'a doctor' means 'some/all doctors'.

5. c. In option **b** the word 'tracing' is used. In common English 'a tracing' is a copy of a picture. 'To trace' can mean 'to find', 'A trace' is what remains when something goes away or disappears as in: 'no trace of the wound remains.'

Exercise 8f

1. Examine the external canal and the eardrum using the auriscope.

2. Prime the syringe with the solution.

3. Place a protective covering over the patient's shoulder.

4. Straighten out the canal by pulling the pinna of the ear gently upwards and backwards.

5. Introduce the fluid through the syringe.

6. Carefully dry the canal after you have examined it to assess the result of the syringing.

Exercise 8g

Beware of the tea cosy

3 000 000 (three million) people are injured in their homes in the UK every year and 4000 (four thousand) of them die. The UK Government has compiled information based on hospital admissions about domestic accidents and a government report is available.

The report says that in 1999 there were 10 773 (ten thousand seven hundred and seventy-three) cases of people treated for accidents caused by socks and tights, 5945 (five thousand nine hundred and forty-five) accidents caused by trousers and 1317 (one thousand three hundred and seventeen) by beanbags. Most of these were falls caused by getting stuck in rushed attempts to get dressed in untidy bedrooms.

Vegetables caused 13 132 (thirteen thousand one hundred and thirty-two) accidents in 1999. The report is not clear about how a vegetable can cause an accident but it is probably because when casualty patients are asked 'what happened?' they say something like, 'it was the mushrooms' and this gets written down as a 'cause'.

1771 (one thousand seven hundred and seventy-one) accidents were caused by leaves, 787 (seven hundred and eighty-seven) by loofahs and sponges and 37 (thirty-seven) by tea-cosies, which is an increase from 20 (twenty) in the previous year. Most of the tea-cosy injuries were scalds caused by picking up a tea-pot by its cosy rather than its handle or tripping up on tea-cosies on slippery kitchen floors.

False teeth caused 933 (nine hundred and thirty-three) accidents, toilet-roll holders 329 (three hundred and twenty-nine), dust-pans 146 (one hundred and forty-six) and bread-bins 91 (ninety-one). A total of 16 662 (sixteen thousand six hundred and sixty-two) people had to go to hospital after accidents with a sofa and 5615 (five thousand six hundred and fifteen) after an accident with a wellington boot.

Exercise 8h

1. c. Neither option **a** nor **b** suggests regularity.
2. a. The word 'some' can refer to a small quantity with the emphasis on 'small'. If you say 'there are *some* paracetamol in this box' with stress on the word 'some', it means there are not many paracetamol in the box.
3. c. 'Somewhat' means 'a little'.
4. a. 'Just fine' means something like 'very good', whereas 'just managing' means surviving but not very well.
5. b. Meanings here depends on the word 'with'. If the report had said 'help *for* Mrs Nolan' the answer would be **c**.
6. b.
7. a. 'Aimless' means without any obvious purpose, without aim.
8. c. 'At other times' means sometimes like this, sometimes like that. In option **c**, 'in turn' has this meaning.

9   **a.**

10   **c.** The District Nurse uses a grammatically passive sentence to suggest that a diagnosis is the responsibility of someone else – in this case a doctor.

Exercise 8i

Mrs Nolan is an <u>elderly</u> woman and, having suffered <u>a</u> stroke, now needs assistance in her <u>daily</u> life. Her husband, who is old and frail, is perhaps <u>finding</u> it difficult <u>to cope</u> at home. Mrs Nolan is often <u>disturbed</u> and <u>distressed</u> and the Day Care staff who know her say that she is either <u>hyperactive</u> or sits <u>lethargically</u>. So far she has not <u>been assessed</u> by a psychiatrist.

Exercise 8j: Further practice

PATIENT ADMISSION FORM

Patient's name
Jacqueline Johnson

Preferred form of address
Jackie

Reason for admission
Superficial burns to L arm, chest & face. Accident in kitchen at home.

Source of information
Mother

Base-line functions	Temp.	Respiration	Circulation
	38.2°c	35/min	128/min

Communication
Says single words, calls urine & stools 'wee-wee'.
Mother says Jackie 'cries a lot'.

Elimination
Wears nappies. Stools strong smelling & slightly discoloured.
Moves bowels 2 × daily

Work and play
Active child. Favourite toy clown 'Ham'.

Eating and drinking
'Good eater'; prefers orange juice to milk.

Chapter Nine

Pain and pain management

Complete this introduction to the subject of pain by filling in the gaps in the text using a choice from each of the brackets:

Describing pain

There are two .... (category, categories, categorise) of pain: acute and chronic. Acute pain .... (subsides, subside, subsidy) as healing takes place and .... (goes, comes, lasts) for a short time, usually for .... (under, not as long, less) than 3 months. Acute pain may be sudden or slow .... (in, on, by) onset and may range from .... (gentle, kind, mild) to severe. In other words it may include .... (anything, all, every) from a pinprick to the pain of an amputation.

Chronic pain is .... (prolonged, prolong, prolongs) for 3 months or longer and ranges from mild to .... (heavy, unkind, severe). If it comes back .... (repetition, repeats, repeatedly), it is called 'recurrent'. To describe levels of pain, hospitals often use a .... (number of, numerical, numbering) scale, e.g. 'pain reduced from 7 to 3'.

The McGill Pain Questionnaire

Describing types of pain can lead to misunderstandings and the McGill Pain Questionnaire was designed to provide vocabulary so that patients can communicate more clearly with nurses and doctors. To describe pain, the McGill Pain Questionnaire uses words like these:

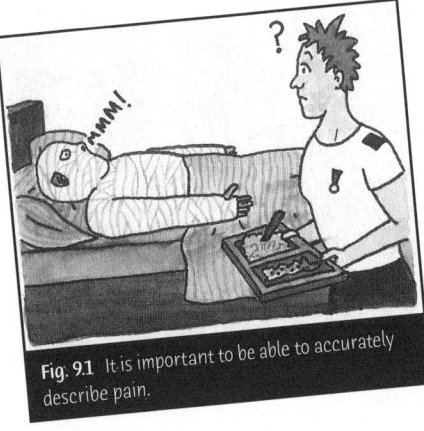

Fig. 9.1 It is important to be able to accurately describe pain.

- **Throbbing.** This means beating repeatedly like a drum.
- **Shooting.** Meaning rushing, like a bullet.
- **Stabbing.** A penetrating pain like a knife being pushed in and taken out.

- **Cramping.** A squeezing, contracting, muscular pain.
- **Gnawing.** Feels like being eaten.
- **Hot, burning.** As if on fire.
- **Aching.** A dull, background pain.
- **Heavy.** A pain which weighs you down.
- **Splitting.** A word often used to describe headaches – as if your head is going to break open.
- **Tiring, exhausting.** A pain that destroys energy.
- **Sickening.** A pain that makes you feel sick.
- **Fearful.** A great pain, central and all-consuming.
- **Punishing, cruel.** A great pain that feels like torture going on and on without relief.

Exercise 9b

From the information above, say which of the following statements are true?

a. Acute pain gets worse as the patient gets better.
b. Acute pain may come on gradually.
c. The higher the number of the pain, the more it hurts.
d. The lower the number, the more it hurts.
e. A pain of '8' is better than a pain of '4'.
f. The McGill Questionnaire describes how much pain a patient feels.

Assessing pain

Mr Morris is 65 years old. He has been admitted to hospital with lung cancer and widespread metastases.

Mr Morris is in a lot of pain and cannot concentrate for long enough to answer many questions. He grimaces frequently (makes facial gestures of pain) and cries. He says things like, 'it hurts, please give me something.'

Location. When the nurse asks him where the pain is, he points to his lower back (site A) and also his right shoulder (site B).

Quality and Intensity. Mr Morris says that the pain at site A is 'an unbearable, gnawing pain' and gets even worse if he coughs. There is a 'sharp' pain in his shoulder (site B) when he coughs.

At the moment, he is taking 90 mg of morphine 4-hourly with 400 mg of ibuprofen 6-hourly.

Here is part of the Pain Assessment Form for Mr Morris.

PAIN ASSESSMENT FORM

Patient's name:
Mr Morris

Diagnosis:
Lung cancer with metastases

Location: (patient or nurse mark drawing)

Intensity – Scale used: 0–10 (10 = worst pain)
Worst pain:
site A = 10 when coughs/site B = 4 when coughs

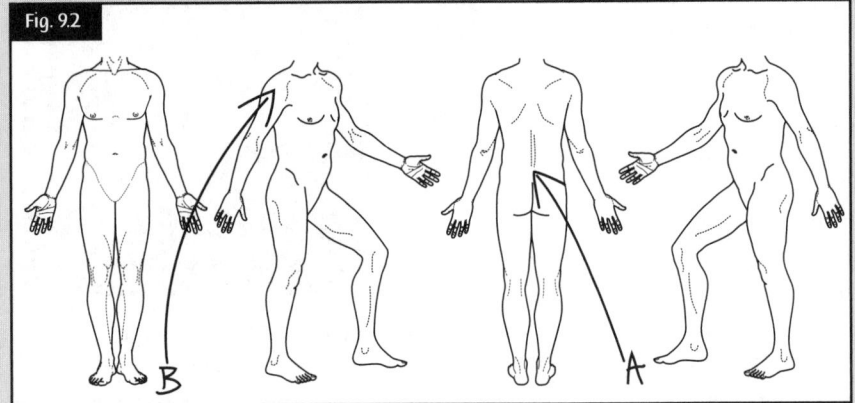

Fig. 9.2

Least pain:
site A = 9 site B = 0

Quality:
A = unbearable gnawing, B = sharp

Manner of expressing pain:
Grimaces and cries. Pain is so bad patient cannot concentrate.

Exercise 9c

Which of the following statements are true?

a. Mr Morris' metastases are localised.
b. He bears the pain silently.
c. The intensity of the pain at site A varies a little.
d. The pain at site A is worse than at site B.
e. He is receiving 90 mg of morphine × 4 every hour.

Now read the next two case histories – of Mr Thompson and Mrs Smith. After each case history, there are some questions to answer followed by a Pain Assessment Form to complete.

CASE HISTORY

Mr Thompson is 45 years old. He had an accident and was admitted to hospital 2 days ago. In surgery he had a splenectomy and a pin was inserted into a fracture of his left femur.

Location and quality of pain. Mr Thompson tells the nurse that it hurts in two places. Site A is on the left side of his abdomen and he describes this pain as 'deep and aching'. Site B is on his left thigh where he describes the pain as 'sharp and throbbing'.

Intensity. The pain is worst at site A (reaching 10) when he coughs. At site B, the pain is worst (reaching 10) when he tries to change his position in bed.

At best, the pain in both sites subsides to 6 when he lies perfectly still. When the pain becomes really bad, Mr Thompson clenches (grips) the side-rails of his bed and grimaces.

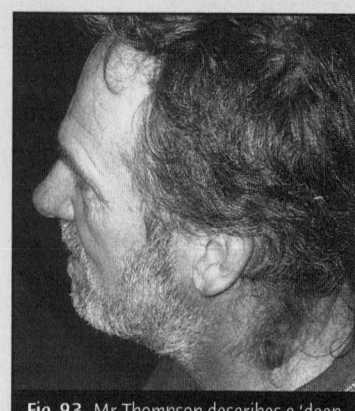

Fig. 9.3 Mr Thompson describes a 'deep aching' pain in his left side and a 'sharp throbbing' pain in his left thigh.

The plan. The patient is receiving 75 mg of pethidine. We will evaluate the patient's response to the pethidine and, if the pain does not subside, then either increase the dose or use an alternative route.

Exercise 9d

1   About Mr Thompson.
The fracture is in:

a. the femur on his left-hand side.
b. the left side of the femur.
c. to the left of the femur.

2   Location and quality of pain.
The pain is:

a. on opposite sides of his body.
b. on the same side but in two different places.
c. in two different places but alike in 'quality'.

3   Intensity of pain.
The pain:

a. varies in intensity.
b. comes and goes.
c. is consistent.

4   The plan
If the pain does not decrease the plan is to:

a. wait and see.
b. increase the dose of painkillers.
c. send the patient to another place for further treatment.

Exercise 9e   **Now fill in the following Pain Assessment Form:**

PAIN ASSESSMENT FORM

Patient's name:
Mr Thompson

Diagnosis:

Location: (patient or nurse mark drawing)

Intensity – Scale used: 0–10 (10 = worst pain)
Worst pain:
Least pain:

Quality:

Manner of expressing pain:

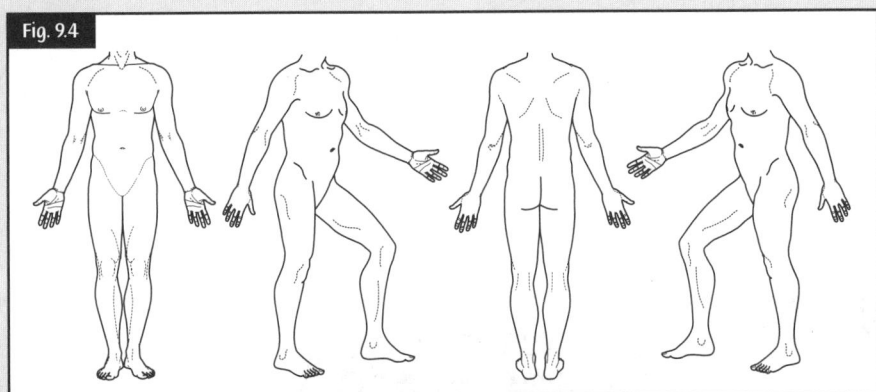
Fig. 9.4

PAIN ASSESSMENT

Mrs Smith is 62 years old. She has breast cancer with bone metastases in the right ribs and lumbar spine. She has arthritis in both her knees and her left shoulder.

Location and quality of pain: There are four main sites of pain.
Site A is just below the patient's ribs on her left hand side.
Site B is in the middle of her lower back.
She describes both A and B as 'constant aching pain'.
Site C is in her left knee.
Site D is on her left shoulder.
She describes both C and D as 'inconsistent and throbbing'.

Intensity: The pain at all the four sites ranges from 3 to 8. At its worst Mrs Smith describes the pain as a 'gnawing, sickening feeling'. However, she says she 'tries to keep going' and she is 'reluctant to bother the nurses'.

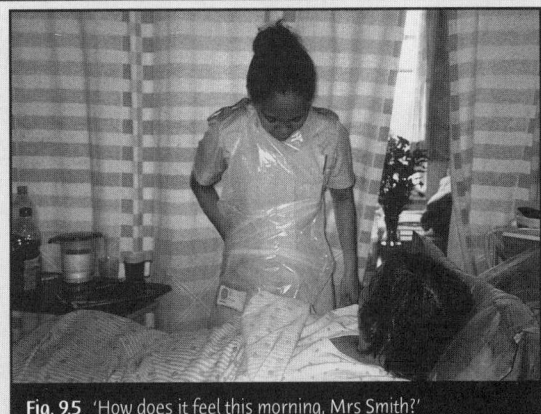
Fig. 9.5 'How does it feel this morning, Mrs Smith?'

Her medication relieves the pain at sites A and B but any movement of her arm makes the pain in her ribs worse, as does sitting upright in a chair. Damp weather makes her shoulders and knees ache more. She falls asleep easily but wakes every 2 or 3 hours because she 'can't get comfortable'.

The Plan: To evaluate the patient's current medication and possibly add non-steroidal anti-inflammatory medication.

Exercise 9f

1   **About Mrs Smith**
The pain from her arthritis is in:

a. a knee.
b. her two knees.
c. knee and shoulders.

2   **Quality of pain**
The pain at sites C and D:

a. comes and goes.
b. is constant.
c. is fading off.

3   **Location of pain**
The pain is:

a. here and there.
b. all over.
c. localised to one side of her body.

Exercise 9g

PAIN ASSESSMENT FORM

Patient's name:
Mrs Smith

Diagnosis:
Breast cancer, bone metastases

Location: (patient or nurse mark drawing with arrows)

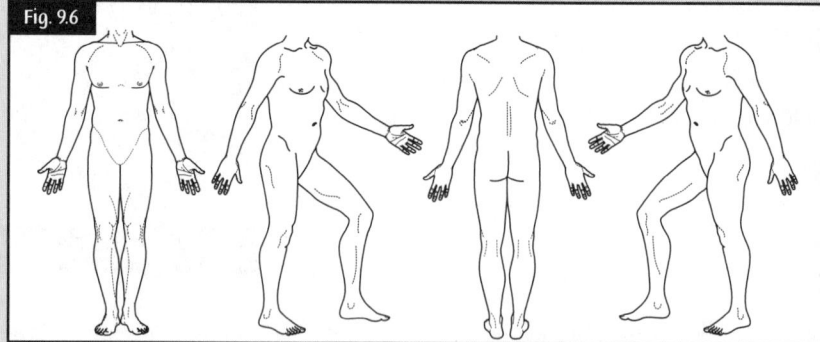

Fig. 9.6

Intensity – Scale used 0–10 (10 = worst pain)
Worst pain:
Least pain:

Manner of expressing pain:

Exercise 9h

The following sentences are about the patients whose details you have just been reading. Fill the spaces in the sentences with vocabulary that has been used in this chapter.

a. Mr Morris .... when the pain gets too much. (meaning: makes a face)

b. Mr Morris is taking 90 mg of morphine orally four .... (meaning: every hour)

c. Mr Thompson has been suffering a .... pain since his operation. (meaning: like a knife)

d. The plan is to see how Mr Thompson .... to pethidine. (meaning: is affected by)

e. Mr Thompson gets .... from the pain by lying perfectly still. (meaning: the pain goes away)

f. The pain in Mrs Smith's shoulder alters in intensity. She describes it as .... (meaning: varying, not always the same)

g. Mrs Smith is shy and doesn't want to .... the nurses. (meaning: cause them trouble)

Exercise 9i

Choose the correct word(s) from the brackets to put into the spaces in the following text:

Mrs Smith has breast cancer with bone metastases. Metastases .... (cause, causes, causing) pain which can .... (ranges, range, ranging) from a .... (loud, splitting, dull) ache .... (from, and, to) a deep oppressive pain.

Often, as with Mrs Smith, the patient .... (expecting, expect, expects) that the nurse will know all .... (of, about, with) her pain. The patient often .... (knows, assumes, says) that the pain is typical and needs no .... (further, farther, far) explanation.

The patient may therefore .... (enjoy, employ, endure) unnecessary pain whilst the nurse is .... (in, with, under) the impression that the pain is .... (in, with, under) control. This means that it is necessary to .... (regular, regulate, regularly) assess a patient's pain and .... (review, reviews, reviewing) the analgesia.

Patients need to .... (informed, be informed, inform) about the cause of their pain and given details about the drugs they are .... (giving, gave, being given). For example they need to be told that constipation is often a .... (side, sides, sided) effect of morphine. Communication .... (between, about, with) patient and medical staff is a very important part of pain control.

Exercise 9j

Read the following article about a controversial issue – the use of an illegal drug to control pain – and answer the questions about the article as you read it.

MAN CLEARED WHO USED CANNABIS AS A PAINKILLER
In June 1998 Colin Davies of Stockport, Manchester was acquitted of
<u>*drugs charges*</u> *when a jury heard he had been growing and smoking*
cannabis to get relief from the pain caused by a broken back.

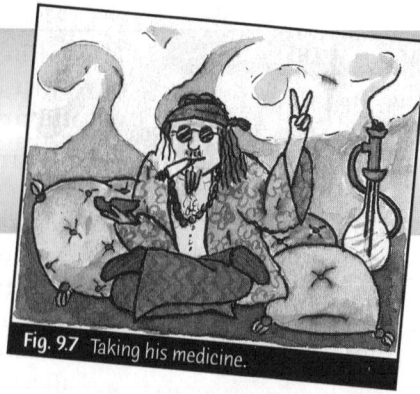

Fig. 9.7 Taking his medicine.

1 'Drugs charges' are:
 a. the cost of drugs.
 b. accusations of criminal offences.
 c. using illegal drugs.

That same year a jury in Warrington also cleared a man who supplied his wife with home-grown cannabis <u>*to ease*</u>
<u>*her pain*</u> *from multiple sclerosis.*

2 Pain that is *eased* is:
 a. pain that comes easily.
 b. pain that increases.
 c. pain that decreases.

Mr Davies suffered severe injuries when he fell 60 feet from a bridge. He smoked four joints a day <u>*to keep the pain*</u>
<u>*at bay*</u> *because the paracetamol and codeine prescribed by doctors did not work. Then he read about cannabis as a*
relief from pain and decided to grow some himself.

3 To 'keep the pain at bay' is to:
 a. lower the pain.
 b. end the pain.
 c. ward the pain off.

The police, <u>*acting on a tip-off,*</u> *raided his home and found cannabis plants in his bedroom. After he was acquitted,*
Mr Davies caused giggles in the court when he asked for his 18 cannabis plants back.

4 To 'act on a tip-off' is:
 a. to do something on a hunch.
 b. to give money for services.
 c. to move on information received.

In a report, the British Medical Association called for greater research into the medical uses of cannabis. It said
that thousands of people are <u>*resorting to the use of cannabis illegally*</u> *because they cannot find conventional relief*
for their symptoms.

5 To 'resort to the use of cannabis illegally' is to:
 a. have no other choice.
 b. take it on holiday.
 c. prefer it to other things.

Labour pain

Mrs Robertson is preparing to give birth and the following notes are entered in her records:

> Mrs Robertson wishes to give birth without drugs. Is apprehensive and agrees to low-dose epidural if pain too much and gas and air ineffective. Wants to feel her legs and push baby out herself.
>
> Mrs R. understands pethidine available but prefers not to use it because of side-effects.

Exercise 9k

Which of the following statements are correct?

a. She will try gas and air before she has the epidural.
b. She believes that pethidine doesn't work.
c. If the epidural doesn't work she will try gas and air.
d. She doesn't want pethidine.
e. She refuses to use pethidine.
f. She wants to feel the baby's legs.
g. She doesn't like what the drug does.
h. Mrs Roberts is not worried.
i. Mrs Roberts wants the baby to push itself out.

Exercise 9l

Fill in the spaces in the following passage by using a word from each bracket.

Pain relief during labour

Pethidine is a .... (derivative, derived, derives) of morphine. It acts .... (in, on, at) the nerve cells in the brain and spinal cord. It is injected into the thigh or bottom and alters a person's .... (perceive, perceptive, perception) of pain. Many women say they find it .... (disoriented, disorientation, disorientating) and .... (uneffective, diseffective, ineffective) as a pain reliever.

An epidural is the most effective method of .... (eradicate, eradicated, eradicating) all sensations of pain. It is a local anaesthetic .... (injected, injection, inject) into the space around the spine. It .... (numbs, numb, numbing) sensation so that the patient doesn't feel .... (a, some, the) contractions. The anaesthetic is then .... (feeding, to feed, fed) continuously via a tube into the epidural space between the spinal cord and the vertebrae in the .... (spine, spinal, spines).

Pethidine crosses the placenta within minutes of .... (given, being gave, being given) and it is .... (necessity, necessarily, necessary) to monitor the fetus electronically to check .... (by, with, for) distress.

Exercise 9m **Say which of the following sentences are grammatically correct.**

a. There's no such thing as a text-book labour.
b. There's no thing as a text-book labour.
c. There is no text-book labour.
d. Contractions aren't constant.
e. Contractions isn't constant.
f. Contractions don't be constant.
g. Contractions peak and died away.
h. Contractions peak then die away.
i. Contractions would peak and then die away.
j. The more it hurts the more closer it is to being over.
k. The more it hurts the closer it is to being over.
l. The most it hurts the closer it is to being over.

Answers and comments on the language

Exercise 9a

There are two <u>categories</u> of pain: acute and chronic. Acute pain <u>subsides</u> as healing takes place and <u>lasts</u> for a short time, usually for <u>less</u> than 3 months. Acute pain may be sudden or slow <u>in</u> onset and may range from <u>mild</u> to severe. In other words it may include <u>anything</u> from a pinprick to the pain of an amputation.

Chronic pain is <u>prolonged</u> for 3 months or longer and ranges from mild to <u>severe</u>. If it comes back <u>repeatedly</u>, it is called 'recurrent'. To describe levels of pain, hospitals often use a <u>numerical</u> scale, e.g. 'pain reduced from 7 to 3'.

Exercise 9b

a. is not true. Acute pain 'subsides' or 'decreases' as the patient gets better.
b. is true. The texts tells us that acute pain may be 'slow in onset'. Note the use of 'onset' meaning 'to come' or 'to appear', e.g. 'the onset of pain may be gradual'.
c. is true. Note the structure of the sentence, very common in describing two things in proportion, e.g. 'the more pain you feel, the less appetite you have.'
d. is not true.
e. is not true. The word 'better' is wrong here. It can be replaced with 'worse' or 'greater', etc. 'The better the pain, the less there is.'
f. is not true. The McGill Pain Questionnaire describes the 'quality' or 'type' of pain rather than the 'degree' or 'intensity' of pain.

Exercise 9c

a. is not true. His metastases are described as 'widespread', whereas 'localised' means limited to certain areas.
b. is not true. Note the use of the word 'bear' meaning 'to carry' the pain or 'to stand' the pain.

c. is true. The pain at site A is always bad but varies from 9 to 10.

d. is true. The pain at site B is only present when the patient coughs.

e. is not true. On the patient's form it says '90 mg of morphine 4-hourly' meaning '90 mg every 4 hours.' '90 mg of morphine × 4 every hour' means 360 mg of morphine every hour.

Exercise 9d

1 a. Mr Thompson's left-hand side femur is the femur on his left side. Option **c** is a place not on the femur but to the left of it. Note the important difference between 'to' (option **c**) and 'on' (option **a**).

2 b. Mr Thompson's pain is on the left side of his abdomen and also on his left thigh.

3 a. The pain is always present and varies from 6 to 10. 'Comes and goes' (option **b**) suggests that sometimes there is no pain. 'Consistent' (option **c**) suggests that the pain is always the same.

4 b. Note the use of 'raise' meaning 'increase'. Note also the use of 'route' in the text meaning 'method of reducing the pain'.

Exercise 9e

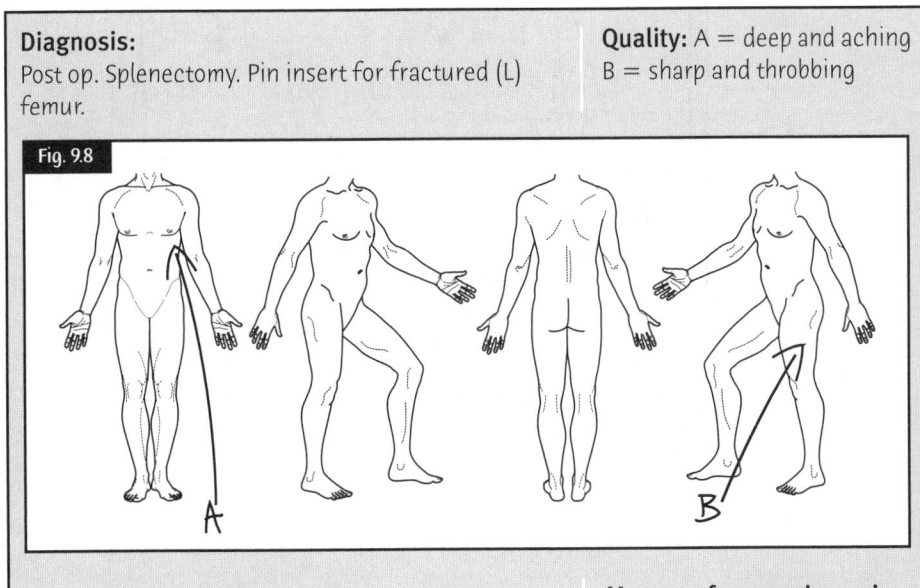

Diagnosis:
Post op. Splenectomy. Pin insert for fractured (L) femur.

Quality: A = deep and aching
B = sharp and throbbing

Fig. 9.8

Worst pain: A = 10 B = 10
Best pain: A = 6 B = 6

Manner of expressing pain:
grimaces & clutches side-rails.

Exercise 9f

1   **b** is the best answer even though she has pain from arthritis in one shoulder as well. Option **c**, 'knee and shoulders', suggests she has pain in one knee and both shoulders.

2   **a.** Mrs Smith says the pain is 'inconsistent', which suggests that it comes and goes. 'Fading off' (option **c**) suggests that the pain is gradually going away.

3   **c.** She has pains in her left shoulder, left knee, and below her ribs on the left-hand side. She also has pain in the middle of her lower back but mostly the pain is on the left side of her body. 'Here and there' (option **a**) is very vague and even suggests that new pains appear in different places at different times.

Exercise 9g

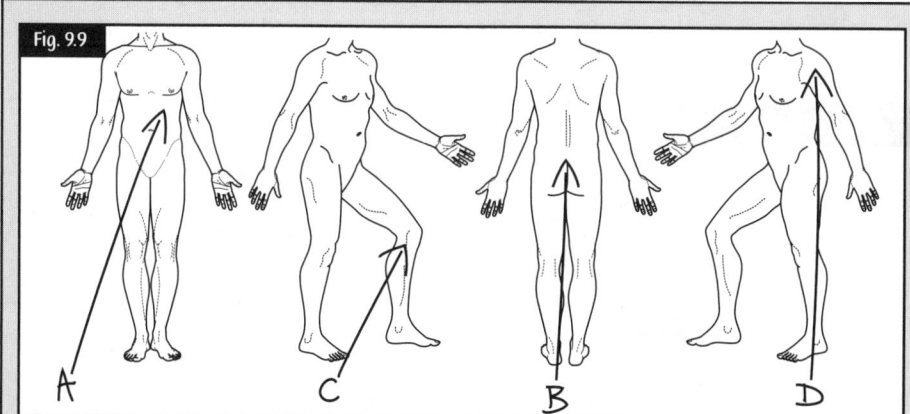

Fig. 9.9

Worst pain: A, B, C, D = 8
Least pain: A, B, C, D = 3

Quality:
A, B = constant, aching C, D = inconsistent, throbbing

Manner of expressing pain:
tries to keep going, stoic, doesn't want to bother nurses.

Exercise 9h

a. Mr Morris <u>grimaces</u> when the pain gets too much.

b. Mr Morris is taking 90 mg of morphine orally four <u>hourly</u>.

c. Mr Thompson has been suffering a <u>stabbing</u> pain since his operation.

d. The plan is to see how Mr Thompson <u>responds</u> to pethidine.

e. Mr Thompson gets <u>relief</u> from the pain by lying perfectly still.

f. The pain in Mrs Smith's shoulder alters in intensity. She describes it as <u>inconsistent</u>.

g. Mrs Smith is shy and doesn't want to <u>bother</u> the nurses.

Exercise 9i

Mrs Smith has breast cancer with bone metastases. Metastases <u>causes</u> pain which can <u>range</u> from a <u>dull</u> ache <u>to</u> a deep oppressive pain.

Often, as with Mrs Smith, the patient <u>expects</u> that the nurse will know all <u>about</u> her pain. The patient often <u>assumes</u> that the pain is typical and needs no <u>further</u> explanation.

The patient may therefore <u>endure</u> unnecessary pain whilst the nurse is <u>under</u> the impression that the pain is <u>under</u> control. This means that it is necessary to <u>regularly</u> assess a patient's pain and <u>review</u> the analgesia.

Patients need to <u>be informed</u> about the cause of their pain and given details about the drugs they are <u>being given</u>. For example they need to be told that constipation is often a <u>side</u> effect of morphine. Communication <u>between</u> patient and medical staff is a very important part of pain control.

Exercise 9j

1 b. If someone is caught 'committing' a crime they are 'arrested' and 'charged'. Later they may be 'tried' in a court.

2 b. You can also say 'pain is relieved' (see Exercise 9h).

3 c. Note that 'to keep something at bay', you 'ward it off', e.g. 'His wife wards off the pain with cannabis.'

4 c. A 'tip' is money you leave a waitress: a 'hunch' (option a) is a suspicion or a 'feeling' or an 'intuition' as in: 'the doctor had a hunch it was cancer'; a 'tip-off' is information given to the police.

5 a. The expression 'a last/final resort' is the last thing you do when you have no more choices left. Note that 'a resort' is somewhere you go for a holiday.

Exercise 9k

Statements **a**, **d** and **g** are correct. All the rest are not true.

Exercise 9l

Pain relief during labour

Pethidine is a <u>derivative</u> of morphine. It acts <u>on</u> the nerve cells in the brain and spinal cord. It is injected into the thigh or bottom and alters a person's <u>perception</u> of pain. Many women say they find it <u>disorientating</u> and <u>ineffective</u> as a pain reliever.

An epidural is the most effective method of <u>eradicating</u> all sensations of pain. It is a local anaesthetic <u>injected</u> into the space around the spine. It <u>numbs</u> sensation so that the patient doesn't feel <u>the</u> contractions. The anaesthetic is then <u>fed</u> continuously via a tube into the epidural space between the spinal cord and the vertebrae in the <u>spine</u>.

Pethidine crosses the placenta within minutes of <u>being given</u> and it is <u>necessary</u> to monitor the fetus electronically to check <u>for</u> distress.

Exercise 9m

The following sentences are grammatically correct:

a.

c. A 'text-book labour' is an 'ideal'. Something which happens in the same way that it is described in a text-book.

d.

h.

i.

k.

Chapter Ten

Mrs Pauline Greene – colostomy

Exercise 10a

VOCABULARY

to siphon (off): to use a tube to extract fluid.

prior to: before.

impacted: very hard – won't move.

dehydration: loss of water.

faeces/stools: waste matter from the bowels. 'Shit', material that is 'defecated'. See 'Euphemisms' in Chapter Seventeen.

nil by mouth: nothing to eat or drink.

purgatives: medicine that causes you to defecate and get rid of material in the stomach.

This text is an introduction to the subject of colostomies and bowel wash-outs. Choose a word from each of the brackets to put in each of the gaps.

A colostomy is an operation which allows .... (faecal, a faeces, faeces) to exit the body either after the rectum .... (has been removed, is removing, removal) or if the rectum has to be bypassed. The surgeon makes an opening .... (in, on, at) the abdomen and .... (attachment, attaches, attaching) the colon to it. A temporary colostomy may be .... (made, did, do) to allow the rectum time .... (to heal, healing, heal) from injury or surgery.

Before .... (making, doing, taking) surgery on the rectum a bowel or rectal wash-out is usually done. This is when fluid is introduced .... (on, via, at) a tube .... (into, by, with) the rectum. The fluid is then .... (siphon, to siphon, siphoned) off in order to help empty the rectum. A bowel wash-out is also .... (do, did, done) before special radiological examinations and in certain cases of impacted faeces.

Mrs Pauline Greene was admitted to the surgical ward on 15 February (15/2) and scheduled for a colostomy on 18 February (18/2). This is her Patient Care Plan:

PATIENT CARE PLAN

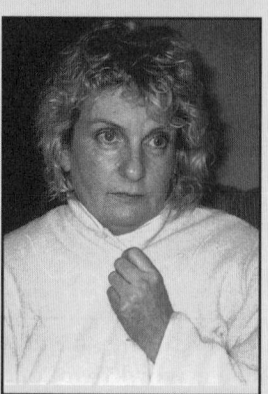

Fig. 10.1 Mrs Greene is worried about her operation.

Patient:
Mrs Pauline Greene.

D.O.B. 7. 5.48

Identified needs/problems:
Prepare for theatre

Eating and drinking:
Potential probs of dehydration due to above

Work and play:
Anxious about effects of stoma on home and social life. To involve family members in care.

Objectives/Goals:
1. minimise risk of post-op. wound infection from bowel contents.
2. allow surgeons clear access to operation site, i.e. free from faeces.
3. complete pre-op. care schedule.
4. encourage patient to voice worries.

Nursing intervention
Rectal wash-out before bedtime for three days (daily)
Purgatives as prescribed
Low-residue light diet 15/2
Fluids only including soup and ice cream 16/2
Clear fluid only 17/2
Nil by mouth from 00.00 hours 18/2
Standard pre-op. procedure.
Ensure variety of acceptable drinks
Mrs Potter (ex-ostomy patient) to visit 16/2
Staff nurse to see Mr and Mrs Greene 17/2 to discuss potential practical probs at home.

Exercise 10b

The Patient Care Plan you have just read covers a period of three days and makes it clear why Mrs Greene is in hospital and what nurses have to do. By using only the information on the Patient Care Plan, say which of the following statements are accurate:

Identified needs/problems

a. Mrs Greene is suffering from dehydration.
b. Mrs Greene is dangerously close to becoming dehydrated.
c. There is a danger that Mrs Greene will become dehydrated.
d. Her preparation for theatre is a cause of dehydration.
e. Mrs Greene is worried about life after the operation.
f. Mrs Greene is anxious about living through the operation.
g. Mrs Greene is anxious about the effects of the stoma on her ability to do sports.
h. Her family should help out with nursing during her stay in hospital.

Objectives/Goals

i. The patient's bowel may infect the wound.
j. The patient has a bowel infection.
k. The surgeon will clear the operation site of faeces.
l. It is best not to upset the patient by discussing the operation.

Nursing intervention

m. Before the operation, Mrs Greene will receive three rectal wash-outs every day.

n. On 15 February, Mrs Greene should have only fluids.

o. She can have ice cream on the day of the operation.

p. It is important to keep Mrs Greene away from ex-ostomy patients.

q. Mrs Potter is a nurse.

r. A member of the medical staff will give Mrs Greene advice after the operation.

Exercise 10c

Here is part of Mrs Greene's Patient Care Plan written out in full sentences. Fill in the gaps in the sentences from the choices in each of the brackets.

Mrs Greene needs .... (to be prepared, prepared, prepare) for theatre on 18 February. The preparation includes .... (reducing, reduction, reduce of) her intake of fluids and food so there is a .... (possible, possibility, possibly) of the patient becoming dehydrated.

It is important .... (to ensure, ensuring, ensured) that the surgeon can have .... (clear, cleared, clearly) access to the operation site and so Mrs Greene's bowel .... (needs, must, have) be clear of all .... (stools, faeces, faecal) matter. Therefore rectal wash-outs should .... (to give, to be given, be given) each evening .... (before, in advance, prior) to the operation. Fluid and food intake .... (needs, should, have) to be reduced to the point where Mrs Greene eats and drinks .... (none, nil, nothing) from midnight on the day .... (of, to, by) the operation.

Mrs Greene is .... (worries, worry, worried) about the consequences of the colostomy and so both she and her husband need an opportunity to discuss things .... (by, with, to) staff and .... (with, for, about) a patient (Mrs Potter) who .... (have had, has had, is having) a colostomy herself.

Exercise 10d

Mrs Greene's Patient Care Plan says that she should receive information and advice about the colostomy she is going to have. Here is some of the information she will be given. First, study the vocabulary list below. Then read the information that comes after it. Choose from a, b or c which is closest in meaning to the words in each paragraph that are underlined.

VOCABULARY

appliance: piece of equipment. In this case the 'appliance' is a bag.

to settle: to go down, decrease in size (swelling).

libido: sex drive.

scarred: wounded and marked after an operation.

intercourse: the sex act.

an erection: an aroused penis.

Sex and the colostomy

1 When you have had a colostomy your stools will pass through the stoma instead of your rectum. Because the stoma has no muscle control, <u>you have to wear an appliance to collect the stools</u>.

a. your faeces goes straight into a bag

b. you must be careful to control your bowels

c. you collect your faeces in a bag after using the toilet

2 The colostomy is usually circular and 3–4 cm across. It may be swollen at first but <u>this will settle in just over a week</u> and other people won't notice it when you are dressed.

a. you won't take any notice of the swelling after a week

b. the swelling will no longer be noticeable after a week

c. after a week you will have got used to the swelling

3 Your general state of health and the stress of the operation may affect your ability to have sex after a colostomy. <u>In theory you can resume sexual activity about six weeks after your operation</u> but in reality many people find that their libido decreases (they lose interest in sex).

a. Six weeks after the operation you will probably want to have sex

b. You should be healed enough to carry on your sex life six weeks after the operation

c. Medical staff will give you permission to have sex after waiting for six weeks after the operation

4 If your rectum has been removed, the tissues nearby may be affected and you may find that having sex hurts so you may need to <u>experiment with different sexual positions</u> until you find one which feels comfortable.

a. have unusual types of sex

b. try sex from different angles

c. have different kinds of sex

5 Some people <u>lose self-confidence</u> after having a colostomy and this affects their sex drive. Men sometimes find it difficult to get an erection. For women, their vagina may be scarred and narrowed, which might make intercourse difficult and painful. Remember that there are other ways of enjoying sex than just intercourse.

a. believe in themselves

b. are afraid of having sex

c. don't feel good about themselves

Exercise 10e

Removing impacted faeces

The following five sentences are instructions to nurses for removing impacted faeces from a patient's rectum. Rewrite the five sentences in such a way that they are as similar as possible in meaning to the originals:

a. The patient should lie on his left side with his knees bent.

It is necessary ....

....

....

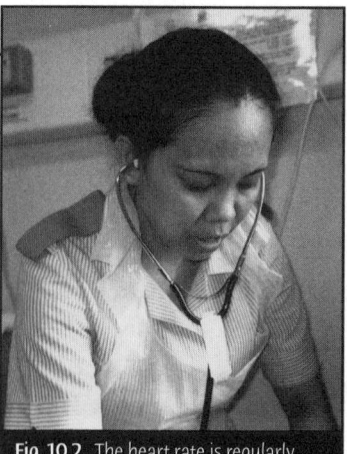

Fig. 10.2 The heart rate is regularly checked for changes in its rhythm.

b. Lay a blanket over the patient's abdomen.
Cover ....
c. Use the index finger to massage around the faecal mass until it is
  loosened.
Loosen ....
d. Check heart rate and stop if changes occur in the rhythm.
Look for any ....
e. Every so often allow the patient to rest.
The patient needs ....

Exercise 10f

Here are extracts from Mrs Greene's records. Answer the questions about each extract by choosing the best answer from a, b and c.

1 The following sentence is in Mrs Greene's Nursing Instructions:
'Address the problem of continuous vomiting and nausea.' What do we
understand from this? That Mrs Greene:
a. is frequently sick and feels sick.
b. is sickly.
c. is sick.

2 The patient was admitted in a poor nutritional state. This indicates that
Mrs Greene:
a. is on a diet.
b. is underweight.
c. can't afford food.

3 The nursing instructions are to give 'third daily changes of the dressing
on her abdominal wound'. This means that the dressing must be
changed:
a. three times a day.
b. 3 × daily.
c. every three days.

4 Under 'Aims' in Mrs Greene's records, is the following entry: 'to
contain effluent and odour.' This means, we aim to:
a. reduce waste matter and smell.
b. dispose of smelly waste matter.
c. keep smells and waste matter in an effective container.

5 Nurses are given the following instructions: 'Apply dressing to the
base of the wound, cover with gauze, and tape to secure.' In other
words, the dressing must be:
a. held in place with adhesive tape.
b. covered with tape.
c. taped with adhesive gauze.

6 A Charge Nurse notes that 'the effluent is proving too thick to drain
adequately and the tubing has twisted in the night cutting off drainage
altogether.' From this we understand that:
a. the tubing has been cut.
b. waste material doesn't flow freely through the tubes.
c. by morning drainage is very slow.

7   Nurses are told that 'overnight drainage of the appliance should be provided to minimise disturbance of the patient.' This means that:

a. Mrs Greene should be enabled to sleep throughout the night.

b. unfortunately the patient will have to be disturbed sometimes during the night, but this should be kept to a minimum.

c. the appliance should be drained nightly.

An adapted drainage system

Here are instructions for an adaptation to Mrs Greene's drainage system. Read them carefully.

THE FOLLOWING EQUIPMENT IS REQUIRED:

One 2-litre plastic milk container with a lid

A length of anaesthetic tubing

A rubber band

Waterproof adhesive tape

Note that the wide bore of the tubing will allow better drainage. The odour will be contained since the unit is sealed.

INSTRUCTIONS:

Secure one end of the plastic tubing with adhesive tape through a hole cut in the lid of the milk container.

Attach the other end to the drainage hole of the fistula appliance by a rubber band and adhesive tape for security.

Remove this system during the day and use a clip thus enabling the patient to move about freely.

Exercise 10g

Say which of the following equipment is needed to make the adaptation:

a. 2 plastic milk containers.

b. A container of milk.

c. A very long tube.

d. A wide tube.

e. Sticky tape.

f. Glue.

Exercise 10h

According to the instructions, say which of the following statements are accurate:

a. The tube must be sealed at one end with adhesive tape.

b. First put the tube in the milk container then put the lid on.

c. Cut a hole in the lid of the milk container.

d. Push the tube through the hole in the lid.

e. Fix the tube to the lid.
f. Attach the other end of the tube to adhesive tape.
g. The system is for night use.
h. Use anaesthetic tubing because it is not very wide.

Exercise 10i

These are the instructions written in another way. Fill in the spaces by choosing a word from the brackets.

Cut a hole ...... (on, at, in) the lid of the milk container and push one ...... (ends, end, part) of the plastic tubing .... (through, past, by) the hole. Fix the tubing firmly .... (on, in, at) place using adhesive tape. Securely connect .... (an, some, the) other end .... (of, from, with) the tubing .... (on, at, to) the drainage hole of the fistula appliance ...... (by, for, to) use ...... (of, for, by) a rubber band as well ...... (at, with, as) adhesive tape.

The system is good for the night time and .... (at, on, during) the day you can take it .... (off, on, of) and close up the drainage system .... (at, under, with) a clip.

Exercise 10j: Further practice

Read this extract from a case history and use it to complete the form that follows.

Mrs Foster went for an operation and when she returned to the ward at 14.00 she was still recovering from the anaesthetic and there was a potential problem of respiratory obstruction. Nurses were instructed to make regular observations of the patient's TPR, to lie the patient in the left lateral position and to take immediate action if her airway became obstructed. Shock could result from decreased volume of circulating blood because of haemorrhage and fluid loss and so it was important to maintain fluid volume. IVI was in progress when she arrived on the ward. Mrs Foster was given 500 ml of dextrox 5% until 15.00 and then 500 ml normal saline solution over the following four hours.

At 17.00, Mrs Foster woke and said she was 'in absolute agony'. The first dose of Omnopon (15 mg) was given and the patient repositioned to keep her as free from pain as possible. Mrs Foster was prescribed 25 mg of Omnopon every 4 hours.

The patient was helped to sit on a bed-pan at 18.00. She was experiencing some discomfort from retention of urine and when this repeated an hour later she was catheterised, producing 200 ml of urine.

Time	Problems/Needs	Nursing Intervention
14.00		
17.00		
18.00		
19.00		

Answers and comments on the language

Exercise 10a

A colostomy is an operation which allows <u>faeces</u> to exit the body either after the rectum <u>has been removed</u> or if the rectum has to be bypassed. The surgeon makes an opening <u>in</u> the abdomen and <u>attaches</u> the colon to it. A temporary colostomy may be <u>made</u> to allow the rectum time <u>to heal</u> from injury or surgery.

Before <u>doing</u> surgery on the rectum, a bowel or rectal wash-out is usually done. This is when fluid is introduced <u>via</u> a tube <u>into</u> the rectum. The fluid is then <u>siphoned</u> off in order to help empty the rectum. A bowel wash-out is also <u>done</u> before special radiological examinations and in certain cases of impacted faeces.

Exercise 10b

a. is not true. Under 'Eating and Drinking' we read that there are 'potential probs' (problems) of dehydration. At the time of writing, the Patient Care Plan, these 'probs' had not arisen.

b. is not true. The words 'potential problems of...' on the Care Plan are a lot less urgent than 'dangerously close to...'

c. is true and the closest in meaning to the original out of **a, b** and **c.** 'There is a danger' suggests that the risk exists but is not great at the moment.

d. is true. This sentence is a warning (it won't necessarily happen).

e. is true.

f. is not true. This sentence says that Mrs Greene is afraid of dying in the operating theatre.

g. is not true. Though a section of the Care Plan is called 'Work and Play', the 'play' part refers to anything which is not work, e.g. home life, watching TV, cooking, going to the cinema, etc. It includes 'games' but does not refer only to games and sports.

h. is not true. Family members will be involved 'in care' but because this comes under 'Work and Play', it refers to life at home not in the hospital.

i. is not true. The danger of infection arises from the contents of the bowel, not the bowel itself.

j. is not true. There is no evidence of this from the Patient Care Plan.

k. is not true. The Patient Care Plan says that this is part of the nurses' task.

l. is not true. The patient is encouraged to 'voice worries'. 'To voice' means to talk about the things which cause anxiety. You 'voice concerns', 'voice fears', 'voice doubts', etc. You let them out.

m. is not true. She will receive one rectal wash-out each day, a total of three before the operation.

n. is not true. ('Low residue diet 15/2')

o. is not true. 'Nil by mouth' from midnight the day of the operation means absolutely nothing to eat and nothing to drink.

p. is not true. In fact the Patient Care Plan says that she should have contact with 'ex-ostomy' patients. Note that medical jargon shortens the word 'colostomy' to 'ostomy'.

q. is not true. Mrs Potter is a patient. She may be a nurse by profession but we don't know that from the Patient Care Plan.

r. is not true. The staff nurse will talk about matters affecting life after the operation but she will do this before Mrs Greene goes for the operation.

Exercise 10c

Mrs Greene needs <u>to be prepared</u> for theatre on 18 February. The preparation includes <u>reducing</u> her intake of fluids and food so there is a <u>possibility</u> of the patient becoming dehydrated.

It is important <u>to ensure</u> that the surgeon can have <u>clear</u> access to the operation site and so Mrs Greene's bowel <u>must</u> be clear of all <u>faecal</u> matter. Therefore rectal wash-outs should <u>be given</u> each evening <u>prior</u> to the operation. Fluid and food intake <u>needs</u> to be reduced to the point where Mrs Greene eats and drinks <u>nothing</u> from midnight on the day <u>of</u> the operation.

Mrs Greene is <u>worried</u> about the consequences of the colostomy and so both she and her husband need an opportunity to discuss things <u>with</u> staff and <u>with</u> a patient (Mrs Potter) who <u>has had</u> a colostomy herself.

Exercise 10d

1　a. To 'control your bowels' (option **b**) is to go to the toilet for yourself. Option **c** creates a picture of a patient first using the toilet then collecting the contents of it.

2　b. Options **a** and **c** suggest that the swelling will be the same but that you will no longer pay it any attention.

3　b. The words 'in theory' suggest that you probably wouldn't want sex even though it would be physically possible.

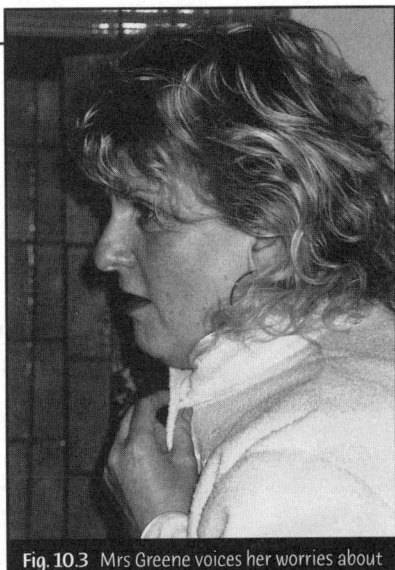
Fig. 10.3 Mrs Greene voices her worries about the colostomy.

4　b. A 'position' is an 'angle' in this case.

5　c. Although 'losing self-confidence' suggests 'being afraid' (option **b**) it is really a more general state in which you have a low opinion of yourself. To 'believe in yourself' (option **a**) is the opposite – it means to *have* self-confidence.

Exercise 10e

a. It is necessary for the patient to lie on his left side with knees bent.
b. Cover the patient's abdomen with a blanket.
c. Loosen the faecal mass by massaging around it with the index finger.
d. Look for any changes in the rhythm of the heart rate and stop if necessary.
e. The patient needs to be allowed to rest every so often.

Exercise 10f

1 a. The difference between options a and c is that a refers to 'vomiting' and c refers to a more general state. 'Sickly' (option b) means 'unhealthy'.

2 b. Option a suggests that Mrs Greene is on a slimmer's diet. Note the difference between being 'on a diet' and 'on a poor diet'. Where the first refers to slimming, the second refers to quality and quantity of food. Option c may be true but we don't know this. A 'poor nutritional state' means 'having eaten very little' so option b is the best choice here.

3 c. 'Every third day' also means the same as 'third daily'.

4 c. 'To contain' is to keep it under control so it doesn't spill over or leak.

5 a. 'To secure' means 'to make it safe so that it won't come undone'.

6 b. There is a difference between 'cut' and 'cut off'. It is the flow of waste matter that is cut off. If the tubes were cut (option a) this would suggest someone has 'severed' them with scissors. Option c is not accurate because the notes tell us that drainage has stopped completely by the morning.

7 a. The main purpose of the adaptation is to give Mrs Greene a chance to sleep at night without having to constantly be getting up. Option c is an instruction to nurses and in fact the purpose of the appliance is to drain at night by itself.

Exercise 10g

d.
e.
Note that 'a container of milk' (option b) refers to something containing milk, whereas a 'milk container' is something that was made to contain milk but is now empty.

The width of the tube (option d) is referred to in the list of equipment as the 'bore'.

Glue (option f) is 'adhesive', but in the list of equipment 'adhesive' is an adjective and refers to sticky tape (option e).

Exercise 10h   The following statements are accurate:

c.

d.

e.

g.

Exercise 10i   Cut a hole <u>in</u> the lid of the milk container and push one <u>end</u> of the plastic tubing <u>through</u> the hole. Fix the tubing firmly <u>in</u> place using adhesive tape. Securely connect <u>the</u> other end <u>of</u> the tubing <u>to</u> the drainage hole of the fistula appliance <u>by</u> use <u>of</u> a rubber band as well <u>as</u> adhesive tape.

The system is good for the night time and <u>during</u> the day you can take it <u>off</u> and close up the drainage system <u>with</u> a clip.

Exercise 10j: Further practice

Time	Problems/Needs	Nursing intervention
14.00	Potential respiratory obstruction	Regular observation of TPR
		Lie in left lateral position
		Respond immediately to obstructed airway
	Possible shock	Maintain fluid vol.
		IVI 500 ml Dextrose 5% until 15.00
		500 ml normal saline until 18.00
17.00	Pain 'absolute agony'	1st dose 15 mg Omnopon
		Reposition patient
		Further 25 mg Omnopon × 4 h
18.00	Discomfort from retention of urine	Bed pan (no urine produced)
19.00	Continued urine retention	Catheterisation (aim to produce 200 ml)

Chapter Eleven

Mr Satawar Hussein – angina

Medical History

Mr Hussein is diagnosed as suffering from angina. The following notes give information about him and his medical history:

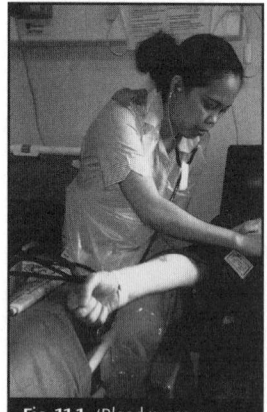

Fig. 11.1 'Blood pressure ranges between 150/90 and 150/100 mmHg.'

> The patient is a 51-year-old, self-employed builder. He is married with two grown-up children. In 1994 he had a heart attack but fully recovered and resumed working. However, a couple of years later Mr Hussein started to suffer increasingly from attacks of breathlessness – at first only when doing physical work but later when resting as well.
>
> A month ago he began to get pains in his arms and chest and suffer from a constant shortness of breath. His GP referred him to hospital for investigation where he was diagnosed as having unstable angina and referred to the cardiac unit where cardiac catheterisation showed major narrowing of his coronary arteries.
>
> The result was coronary bypass surgery two days ago to improve the blood supply to his heart and he is now recovering from the operation. He accepts the situation and is optimistic and cheerful, but he is anxious about post-operation progress and concerned about losing his HGV licence as a result of his illness.
>
> Problems
>
> He has not slept well since coming to hospital. He has nightmares and usually wakes at 2.00 and dozes on and off until 7.00, then feels tired for most of the day.
>
> He has sternal wound pain which he describes as 'stabbing' and 'burning' – point 5 at best and 8/9 at worst (on a scale of 1–10). There are high levels of muscular aches and pains all over his arms and legs. These pains he describes as 'throbbing' – point 4 at best and 8 at worst. Lack of sleep increases his sensitivity to pain.
>
> Blood pressure is in the range of 150/90–150/100 mmHg. There is a potential for post-operative wound infection.
>
> Aims
>
> Post-operative wounds are expected to be healed and free from infection within 6–12 weeks.
>
> Nursing instructions
>
> The patient should receive analgesia after 22.00 in order to provide longer relief from discomfort after lights are turned out. He should be given as many pillows as he wants and noise in the ward should be reduced to a minimum. He should be allowed time for sleep periods during the day. The patient should have two showers daily when skin antiseptic should be applied. Avoid salt in food.

Exercise 11a

1   A 'shortness of breath' is:
a. when you breathe hard.
b. when it is hard to breathe.
c. when you pant.

2   To 'suffer increasingly from attacks of breathlessness' is:
a. to have more and more attacks of breathlessness.
b. to have worse and worse attacks of breathlessness.
c. to start getting attacks of breathlessness.

3   Mr Hussein is 'anxious about post-operative progress.'
This means:
a. he is concerned about what his life is going to be like in the future.
b. he is worried about how he is getting on.
c. he thinks he's going to die.

4   To 'doze on and off' is to:
a. repeatedly fall deeply asleep then wake.
b. sleep deep then shallow, then deep, then shallow and so on.
c. have shallow sleep that comes and goes.

5   'Lack of sleep increases his sensitivity to pain' means:
a. he can't sleep because of the pain.
b. he needs to sleep to avoid the pain.
c. not being able to sleep means he feels the pain more.

6   'Reduce noise in the ward to a minimum' means:
a. make as little noise as possible.
b. make no noise at all.
c. maintain silence at all times.

7   'He is concerned about losing his HGV licence' means:
a. he is worried because he can't find his licence.
b. he may have forgotten how to drive a lorry.
c. he may be disqualified from driving lorries.

Exercise 11b

Say which of the following statements are true:
a. Mr Hussein has had three operations within the last twelve months.
b. The patient drives a lorry.
c. The patient is a lorry driver.
d. Mr Hussein was brought to hospital by his GP.
e. Mr Hussein is unstable.
f. Mr Hussein has an unstable condition.
g. Mr Hussein has disturbed nights.
h. The patient should take analgesic in the early evening.
i. The patient should lie flat in bed.
j. The patient should have a shower once every two days.

Exercise 11c

The text that follows is about wound-dressing following the kind of surgery Mr Hussein has received. Put the following prepositions into the spaces in the text:

into, to, after, or, by, when, through

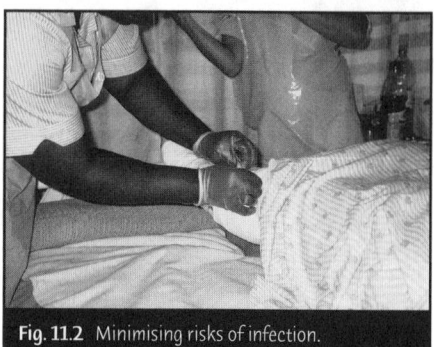

Use aseptic wound dressing .... reduce any potential problems .... the introduction of pathogenic microorganisms .... the body .... the effectiveness of the natural body defences is reduced. Use sterile equipment, lotions and dressings so that the risk of contamination .... airborne pathogenic microorganisms is kept .... a minimum. Aseptic wound-dressing procedures are used .... an invasive procedure such as catheterisation.

Fig. 11.2 Minimising risks of infection.

Exercise 11d

This is Mr Hussein's Patient Care Plan. There are spaces in it and you must fill in the spaces by choosing the best option from the choices provided.

PATIENT CARE PLAN	

Patient: **D.O.B.**
Mr Satawar Hussein   5.5.51

Next of kin:
Mrs S. Hussein (wife)

Identified needs/problems
1. ....
2. ....

Number 1
Either: a. Possible post-op. infection.
  Or: b. Infection post op.
  Or: c. Reduce post-op. infection.

Number 2
Either: a. Localised pain ranging from worst 4 to best 8.
  Or: b. Pains all over body ranging from worst 4 to best 8
  Or: c. Throbbing pain all over best 4, worst 8.

Eating and drinking
Restricted diet

Work and play
....

Either: a. Patient concerned about lost HGV licence.
  Or: b. Patient concerned about losing HGV licence.
  Or: c. Patient has lost HGV licence & concerned about post-op. progress.

Sleep
Has trouble sleeping and wakes at night at 2.00. Has bad dreams.

Objectives/goals
1. ....
2. Improve sleep to aid recovery process and relieve pain at night.
Either: a. Post-op. wounds are healed & free from infection.
  Or: b. Post-op. wounds will heal between 6 & 12 weeks.
  Or: c. Post-op. wounds to heal within 6–12 weeks.

Nursing intervention
1. ....
2. ....
3. ....
4. Reduce noise in ward to min. poss.

Number 1
Either: a. 2 showers twice a day – use antiseptic.
  Or: b. Daily, 2 showers plus antiseptic.
  Or: c. Shower with antiseptic twice a day.

Number 2
Either: a. Minimum salty food.
  Or: b. No salt.
  Or: c. Take out salt from food.

Number 3
Either a. Patient to have analgesia at 22.00.
  Or: b. Analgesics administered no later than 22.00.
  Or: c. Give analgesics later than 22.00.

Exercise 11e   The following text is about the treatment of angina. Fill in the gaps using a word(s) in the brackets.

Patients with angina can .... (suffer, get, make) relief from the symptoms by .... (getting, doing, taking) nitrate drugs which work very quickly. They are available in tablet .... (design, form, structure) or skin patches.

Because the body learns how .... (toleration, to tolerate, tolerance) the drugs, after a while they no longer work so patients need to have .... (free nitrate, nitrate-free, without nitrate) periods. The disadvantage of nitrates is that they can .... (cause, make, create) headaches, puffiness and .... (swelling, swollen, swell) of ankles and legs.

Beta-blockers are also .... (taken, brought, given) to patients with angina, which make their heart beat slower. However, these can cause patients' .... (extreme, extremely, extremities) to become cold and should not be .... (taken, given, prescribed) by asthmatics, diabetics and people with .... (poorly, poor, the poor) circulation.

Exercise 11f   Look at the following list of words and put the appropriate ones into the spaces in the sentences about angina that come after the list. Each word will have to be changed in some way to make each sentence grammatically correct. (Some sentences have more than one answer.)

bother

squeeze

trigger

breathless

narrow

grip

acceleration

block

a. Patients with coronary heart disease describe angina as a .... pain in the chest.
b. It feels as if your chest is being .... or crushed.
c. The pain is caused by .... in the arteries.
d. You can be .... by angina when doing hard physical work.
e. Angina can also be .... by intense emotion, a heavy meal or even a cold wind.
f. Along with the pain may come ....
g. The main problem that causes angina is .... of the blood vessels.
h. Normally this happens with age but it is .... by smoking.

Exercise 11g

These are questions which you might ask a patient suffering from pains in the chest. Say which ones are grammatically correct:

1
a. Are you high blood pressure?
b. Do you high blood pressure?
c. Do you have high blood pressure?

2
a. Do anyone in your family has heart disease?
b. Has anyone in your family do heart disease?
c. Does anyone in your family have heart disease?

3
a. Do you smoke?
b. Do you smoking?
c. Are you smoker?

4
a. What age you are?
b. What's your age?
c. What are your age?

5
a. How long you have this pain?
b. How long is this pain?
c. How long have you had this pain?

Exercise 11h

Fill in the spaces in the following text which is about tests to do with angina using the correct word(s) from each of the brackets.

There are a number of tests that can .... (perform, performed, be performed) to get more information about .... (a patient's, patient's, patients) angina. The first .... (to do, is, are) an electro-cardiogram (ECG). This is normally done .... (during, at, whilst) the patient is .... (suffers, suffer, suffering) from a chest pain.

There is also something called a stress test which is .... (perform, done, be performed) while the patient walks on .... (a, the, some) treadmill so that it is possible to see how the heart is .... (perform, performance, performing) when the patient .... (exercising, exercises, exercise).

X-rays of the heart taken .... (in front and behind, before and after, early and late) exercise can show if an area of the heart is .... (no, none, not) getting enough blood. If this happens it may mean that arteries supplying blood to the heart .... (are, is, be) blocked.

Another test is cardiac .... (catheterisation, catheterise, catheter). This is a test .... (in which, which, that) a long thin tube is inserted through the artery in an arm or a leg and then .... (to be guided, guided, guides) into the heart. Dye is then injected .... (onto, at, into) the arteries around the heart and the heart is then .... (X-ray, to X-ray, X-rayed) to see if any of the arteries are blocked.

Exercise 11i: Further practice

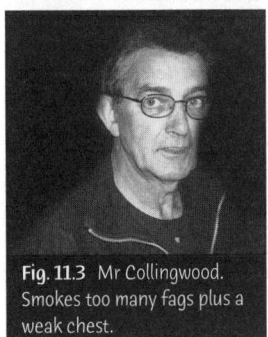

Fig. 11.3 Mr Collingwood. Smokes too many fags plus a weak chest.

Use the following information to complete the form that comes after it.

Mr John Collingwood is 52 years old. He lives with his wife Mary. He has had chronic bronchitis since he was 25 and he had pneumonia in childhood. He smokes 30 cigarettes a day. He has a morning cough and wheeziness as he breathes and gets a lot of chest infections. He has a high carbohydrate intake and drinks a lot of beer.

Over the past two weeks, Mr Collingwood has had two severe asthma attacks and was admitted to hospital when the third attack did not respond to his usual treatment. He was diagnosed as 'severe acute asthma'.

On admission the patient had to sit upright in order to be able to breathe and said he found it difficult to sleep when lying flat. He therefore uses at least two pillows. The patient is very frightened of dying and needs constant reassurance.

PATIENT ASSESSMENT RECORD

Patient's name:

Age:

Form of address:

Next of kin:

Relevant medical history:

Medical diagnosis:

Patient's feelings and expectations related to present illness:

Eating and drinking:

Breathing:

Sleeping:

Answers and comments on the language

Exercise 11a

1　b. 'A shortness of breath' is the same as 'breathlessness' (see Question 2). 'Panting' (option c) is the rapid breathing that happens after running or other intense physical exertion.

2　a. Here, the word 'increasingly' describes 'to suffer' – in other words, Mr Hussein has more and more attacks rather than worse and worse attacks. If you wanted to say that the attacks get worse and worse you could say: 'to suffer from attacks of increasing breathlessness'.

3 b. 'Post-operative progress' is what happens to your body after an operation. 'Getting on' (option **b**) is commonly used to mean 'progress' as in: 'how are you getting on?'

4 c. 'To doze' is to sleep in a shallow way. 'On and off' means 'sometimes and sometimes not.'

5 c. Note the expression 'lack of sleep'. 'Lack of' means 'without'. It can be used as a verb, as in: 'he lacks sleep'.

6 a. 'A minimum' is the smallest possible. There is also a verb 'to minimise' meaning to make as small as possible, e.g. 'to minimise the noise in the ward', meaning, 'to decrease the noise in the ward to the lowest possible.'

7 c. HGV stands for 'Heavy Goods Vehicle', which is a lorry weighing over 5 tons. 'To lose your licence' is to have it taken away, which means the same as 'to be disqualified from driving'.

Exercise 11b

a. is not true. Mr Hussein has had 1 operation – coronary bypass.

b. is true.

c. is not true. Note the difference between **b** and **c.** Mr Hussein is a builder who drives a lorry.

d. is not true. To be brought to hospital would involve his GP physically taking him. His GP 'sent' him to hospital. The differences between 'send', 'take' and 'bring' often cause confusion.

e. is not true. The word 'unstable' in a sentence like this usually refers to an emotional/mental condition.

f. is true. The angina is classified as 'unstable' and the word here refers to the angina, not to the patient as it does in **e.**

g. is true. 'Disturbed' here refers to sleep. If he keeps waking up or can't sleep or has nightmares, then his nights are described as 'disturbed'.

h. is not true. The Nursing Instructions are to give Mr Hussein analgesics late in the evening/at night so that his nights might be pain-free.

i. is not true.

j. is not true. The Nursing Instructions say; 'two showers daily' meaning 'every day have two showers.'

Exercise 11c

Use aseptic wound dressing <u>to</u> reduce any potential problems <u>through</u> the introduction of pathogenic microorganisms <u>into</u> the body <u>when</u> the effectiveness of the natural body defences is reduced. Use sterile equipment, lotions and dressings so that the risk of contamination <u>by</u> airborne pathogenic microorganisms is kept <u>to</u> a minimum. Aseptic wound dressing procedures are used <u>after</u> an invasive procedure such as catheterisation.

Exercise 11d

PATIENT CARE PLAN

Patient:
Mr Satawar Hussein

D.O.B.
5.5.51

Next of kin:
Mrs S. Hussein (wife)

Identified needs/problems
1 a. possible post-op. infection.
2 c. throbbing pain all over
best 4 to worst 8.

Eating and drinking
Restricted diet

Work and Play
b. patient concerned about losing
HGV licence.

Sleep
Has trouble sleeping and wakes at
night at 2.00. Has bad dreams.

Objectives/goals
c. Post-op. wounds to heal within
6–12 weeks.
Improve sleep to aid recovery
process and relieve pain at night.

Nursing intervention
1 b. Daily, 2 showers plus
antiseptic.
2 b. No salt.
3 c. Give analgesics later than
22.00.
4 reduce noise in ward to min. poss.

Exercise 11e

Patients with angina can <u>get</u> relief from the symptoms by <u>taking</u> nitrate drugs which work very quickly. They are available in tablet <u>form</u> or skin patches.

Because the body learns how <u>to tolerate</u> the drugs, after a while they no longer work so patients need to have <u>nitrate-free</u> periods. The disadvantage of nitrates is that they can <u>cause</u> headaches, puffiness and <u>swelling</u> of ankles and legs.

Beta blockers are also <u>given</u> to patients with angina, which make their heart beat slower. However, these can cause patients' <u>extremities</u> to become cold and should not be <u>taken</u> by asthmatics, diabetics and people with <u>poor</u> circulation.

Exercise 11f

a. Patients with coronary heart disease describe angina as a <u>squeezing/gripping</u> pain in the chest.
b. It feels as if your chest is being <u>gripped/squeezed</u> or crushed.
c. The pain is caused by <u>blockage(s)</u> in the arteries.
d. You can be <u>bothered</u> by angina when doing hard physical work.
e. Angina can also be <u>triggered</u> by intense emotion, a heavy meal or even a cold wind.
f. Along with the pain may come <u>breathlessness</u>.
g. The main problem that causes angina is <u>narrowing/blocking</u> of the blood vessels.
h. Normally this happens with age but it is <u>accelerated</u> by smoking.

Exercise 11g

The following questions are grammatically correct:

1 c. Do you have high blood pressure?
2 c. Does anyone in your family have heart disease?
3 d. Do you smoke?
4 e. What's your age?
5 f. How long have you had this pain?

Exercise 11h

There are a number of tests that can <u>be performed</u> to get more information about <u>a patient's</u> angina. The first <u>is</u> an electrocardiogram (ECG). This is normally done <u>whilst</u> the patient is <u>suffering</u> from a chest pain.

There is also something called a stress test which is <u>done</u> while the patient walks on <u>a</u> treadmill so that it is possible to see how the heart is <u>performing</u> when the patient <u>exercises</u>.

X-rays of the heart taken <u>before and after</u> exercise can show if an area of the heart is <u>not</u> getting enough blood. If this happens it may mean that arteries supplying blood to the heart <u>are</u> blocked.

Another test is cardiac <u>catheterisation</u>. This is a test <u>in which</u> a long thin tube is inserted through the artery in an arm or a leg and then <u>guided</u> into the heart. Dye is then injected <u>into</u> the arteries around the heart and the heart is then <u>X-rayed</u> to see if any of the arteries are blocked.

Exercise 11i. Further practice

Patient:
John Collingwood

Age:
52

Form of address:
Mr

Next of kin:
Mrs Mary Collingwood (wife)

Relevant medical history:
Chronic bronchitis (27 years)
2 recent attacks asthma
Pneumonia when child
Frequent chest infections

Medical diagnosis:
Severe acute asthma

Patient's feelings and expectations related to present illness:
Is afraid of dying and needs comforting

Eating and drinking:
Drinks a lot (beer)
A lot of carbohydrates

Breathing:
Smokes 30 cigarettes per day
Morning cough, wheezy chest
Must sit upright to breathe

Sleeping:
Difficulty sleeping flat – needs two pillows.

Chapter Twelve

Mr Bob Jameson – dehydration

Mr Jameson is suffering from severe dehydration. This is his Patient Care Plan:

PATIENT CARE PLAN

Patient:
Mr Robert Jameson

Next of kin:
Mr Leroy Jameson (son)

Needs/problems
Dehydration, inadequate fluid intake, dry, dehydrated skin.
Dry lips, coated tongue.
Decreased urinary output.

Objectives/goals
Adequate hydration.
Moist lips & tongue.
Urinary output of at least 2000 ml per day. Urine concentration (specific gravity) 1.010–1.025.
Daily bowel action.

Nursing intervention
At least 3000 ml daily.
  0800–1600 : 1500 ml
  1600–2200 : 1000 ml
  2200–0800 : 500 ml.

Sit patient well up before giving drink.
Offer drinks hourly (prefers tea/lemon – does not like coffee)
Mouth care 4-hourly.
Observe & record output. Report inadequate output.
Test urine for specific gravity, report abnormal findings.
Record bowel actions. Add bran to cereal. Plenty fruit.

Exercise 12a

From your reading of Mr Jameson's Patient Care Plan, say which of the following statements are true:

a. Leroy Jameson is Robert Jameson's sibling.

b. Mr Jameson is a drinker.

c. Mr Jameson needs to drink.

d. The specific gravity of Mr Jameson's urine is between 1.010 and 1.025.

e. Anything out of the ordinary should be recorded.

f. Mr Jameson should avoid too much fruit.

Exercise 12b   **Which sentence out of a, b or c is grammatically correct?**

1   a. Mr Jameson has a dehydration.
b. Mr Jameson is dehydrated.
c. Mr Jameson is a dehydrate.

2   a. He doesn't produce enough urine.
b. He isn't produces enough urine.
c. He doesn't produce not enough urine.

3   a. The goal is an increase urine production.
b. The goal is to increase urine production.
c. The goal is increase urine production.

4   a. His urine needs to test specific gravity.
b. His urine need to be tested for specific gravity.
c. The specific gravity of his urine needs to be tested.

5   a. The patient should sit well up before drinking.
b. The patient should well sit up before drinking.
c. The patient should sit up before drinks well.

6   a. His output of urine needs to be recorded.
b. His output of urine must to be recorded.
c. His output of urine should to be recorded.

Exercise 12c   **Here is the information in the Patient Care Plan written out in full. Fill in the spaces with a word from each of the brackets:**

Mr Jameson is taking in a(n) .... (not sufficient, non-sufficient, insufficient) quantity of fluid which is causing his skin ....
.... (is becoming, became, to become) dry. It is necessary to ....
(ensure, sure, assure) the patient takes in .... (least, minimum, at least) 3000 ml of fluid every day and nurses must .... (sat, seat, sit) the patient upright before giving him an .... (hourly, every hour, each hour) drink.

The aim is to get Mr Jameson to produce more than 2000 ml of urine .... (all, every, most) day. It is .... (necessary, necessity, necessarily) to measure the specific gravity of his urine. Any abnormalities out ....
(by, in, of) the range of 1.010–1.025 .... (need, have, should) be reported.

Keep the patient's mouth, teeth and dentures .... (clean, cleaned, to clean). Ensure oral hygiene is done .... (each, all, every) four hours in order .... (encouraging, encouragement, to encourage) a flow of saliva to keep the patient's oropharyngeal muscles healthy.

Exercise 12d   **Rewrite the following sentences so that the words in brackets appear at the beginning of each of your new sentences. The first one is done for you:**

Once the urine sample has been obtained it should be tested immediately. (You should...).

Answer: You should test the urine sample immediately you have obtained it/it has been obtained.

a. Inaccurate results are often obtained if the urine is left exposed to the air. (You may get...)

b. Fresh urine from a healthy person should not have an unpleasant smell. (A healthy person's...)

c. Decomposing urine smells like ammonia. (A smell like ammonia...)

d. Diabetes mellitus may be indicated by sweet-smelling urine. (Sweet-smelling urine...)

e. Urine that smells of fish may indicate infection of the urinary system. (A urinary infection...)

f. Dehydration is indicated by dark-coloured urine. (Dark-coloured...)

g. The concentration of substances dissolved in the urine is measured by specific gravity. (Specific gravity...)

h. The normal range for the specific gravity of urine is between 1.005 and 1.025. (A range of 1.005 to 1.025...)

i. Little information is got from a single measurement. (A single measurement...)

j. A low specific gravity indicates renal damage or diabetes insipidus. (Diabetes insipidus...)

Exercise 12e

The text that follows is advice to nurses about getting urine samples. Fill in the spaces using a word from each of the brackets:

How to get urine for testing

You should aim for a 'clean catch' urine sample which is .... (free from, free to, freed by) contaminants. In the case of men, the head of the penis .... (has, should, must to) be wiped clean. Women .... (will, might, should) first wash the area between the lips of the vulva with .... (soap, soaped, soapy) water .... (Using, Used, Use) a clean container and catch .... (into, during, between) 30–60 ml of urine after .... (allow, allowed, allowing) the first small amount to fall into the toilet .... (bowl, basin, pot) so that you get your sample from .... (middle of, central, mid) stream.

Exercise 12f

Mr Jameson's condition does not improve and a few days after the above entries were made in his Patient Care Plan, a Staff Nurse writes the following comments about him:

Patient refuses drinks – increasingly unco-operative. Urine output now < 1000 ml (16/9) – dark colour. Specific gravity test = 1.035 (cause for concern). No bowel action recorded (16/9).

Write out these comments in full sentences by rearranging the groups of words below so that they make meaningful sentences:

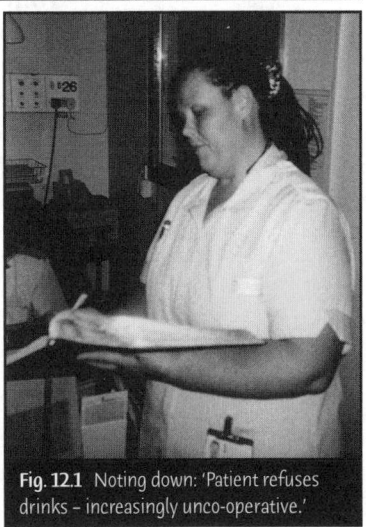

Fig. 12.1 Noting down: 'Patient refuses drinks – increasingly unco-operative.'

1 the patient/is/Mr Robert Jameson/unco-operative/becoming

2 his dehydration is getting worse/that are offered to him/drinks/he is refusing/and as a consequence/

3 dark-coloured urine/have dropped to a worrying 1.035/on 16 September/than 1000 ml of/he produced less/and the results of the test of specific gravity

4 had no/on 16 September/also he has/bowel movement.

Exercise 12g

Study the following vocabulary and adapt the words if necessary to fit the text which comes afterwards. The text gives further information about dehydration:

VOCABULARY

to lag behind: to be second, to come afterwards, to be late.

dizzy: the feeling in your head when you become unbalanced.

to flush: to redden in the face and feel suddenly warm.

to consume: to eat or drink.

to exhale: to breathe out (to 'inhale' is to breathe in).

caffeine: the stimulant in coffee/tea/Coca-Cola, etc.

to pay attention: to notice and respond to.

profuse: a lot.

A healthy adult will lose something like 2.4 litres of fluid every day in the form of sweat, urine, ... air and bowel movements. The feeling of thirst will normally .... the need to drink because it may take some time for your body .... to the sensation of thirst.

If it is left without fluid for too long, the body will start to show signs of dehydration such as feelings of .... The body will become .... and start sweating .... There is danger when the body actually *stops* sweating.

The best solution to dehydration is simply ...... plenty of water. Soft drinks manufacturers spend huge quantities of money on persuading us to buy their soft drink products but in fact the best choice is water. ...... drinks as well as alcohol will in fact increase dehydration because they increase urine output.

Exercise 12h

As you know, patients like Mr Jameson who refuse help from nursing staff are quite common. These people are described in the sentences below. Rewrite each of the sentences beginning with the words in brackets, the first is done for you as an example. (Source: J.E. Groves. Taking care of the hateful patient. N. Engl. J. Med. 1978; 278:883–887.)

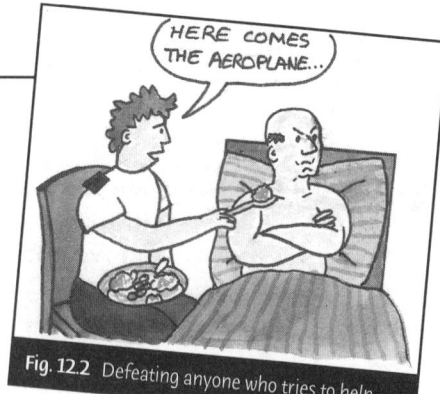

HERE COMES THE AEROPLANE...

Fig. 12.2 *Defeating anyone who tries to help.*

Some patients may reject help because they want to have control over medical staff. (A patient who wants...)

Answer: A patient who wants to control medical staff may reject help.

a. These patients do not believe that any treatment will help them. (These patients believe...)

b. They get satisfaction from reporting the failure of treatments to medical staff. (Telling medical staff that...)

c. It is said that these patients do not want relief from any illness but rather a long-term relationship with a medical practitioner. (These patients are looking more...)

d. Practitioners are often made to feel guilty and inadequate when dealing with patients like these. (Patients like these will often...)

e. These patients defeat anyone who tries to help. (Anyone who...)

f. Only their own self-destruction will satisfy them. (They get satisfaction...)

g. The advice is not to abandon these patients but to work with them like patients with terminal cancer. (These patients should not...)

Exercise 12i **The following sentences are about diarrhoea and dehydration. Say which of a, b or c can replace the part of each sentence which is in brackets.**

1 (An abnormal fluidity of) faeces is a characteristic of diarrhoea.
a. Easy passing of
b. A lot of water in the
c. Extremely runny

2 A patient with diarrhoea (has an abnormal amount of faecal evacuations.)
a. produces a lot of abnormal faeces.
b. goes to the toilet a lot.
c. passes large quantities of stools each time.

3 (Watery) stools are passed at least three times a day.
a. Runny
b. Soft
c. Wet

4 Passing large quantities of (formed) stools is not diarrhoea.
a. hard
b. normal
c. small

5 It is not the quantity but the (consistency) that is important.
a. quality
b. thickness
c. degree of firmness

6 Diarrhoea is dangerous because it causes a rapid (depletion) of water and sodium which are both necessary for life.
a. reduction
b. absence
c. emptying

7 Dehydration is often caused by (persistent) diarrhoea that lasts fourteen days or more.
a. continual
b. regular
c. frequent

8 Early features of dehydration include dry mouth, thirst, weak pulse and (loss of skin elasticity).
a. dull, unhealthy looking skin.
b. flaky, dry skin.
c. when you pinch the skin it goes back slowly.

9 Oral rehydration therapy (ORT) does not stop the diarrhoea but it does (replace) lost fluids and essential salts.
a. put back
b. put in
c. put by

10 (Glucose added to) ORS solution, enables the intestine to absorb fluid and salts more efficiently.
a. Extra glucose in
b. Adding glucose to
d. The adding of more glucose to

11 ORT is normally (an effective) treatment for patients suffering from acute watery diarrhoea.
a. a useful
b. an adequate
c. a complete

Exercise 12j

Fill in the spaces in the following passage about oral rehydration therapy with the correct word from the brackets.

You can use ...... (the, some, a) simple salt/sugar solution for ORT. Mix .... (the, some, a) level teaspoon of salt with 8 .... (flat, smooth, level) teaspoons of sugar in .... (the, some, a) litre of drinking water.

It is a good idea to use molasses or .... (the, a, some) other form of unrefined sugar because unrefined sugar contains .... (more, most, very) potassium than white sugar. Do not use .... (too, to, two) much salt because .... (in, at, on) some cases, salt can cause convulsions. Too .... (less, small, little) salt does no ...... (harm, danger, risk) but it is .... (less, under, small) effective ...... (to, in, at) preventing dehydration. As a rule of .... (finger, thumb, hand) for the amount of salt to use in the solution, ... (they, it, them) should taste ...... (no, less, un-) saltier than tears.

Answers and comments on the language

Exercise 12a

a. is not true. 'Sibling' means brother or sister. 'Spouse' is also a common word used on official documents, forms and records which means 'husband' or 'wife'.

b. is not true. 'A drinker' in UK English is generally a person who drinks a lot of alcohol. 'A drink' can often refer to alcohol in UK English as in: 'he drinks a lot'. 'Drink to someone' is to toast (celebrate) them. 'Have a drink on me' can mean 'accept this money' (as a tip).

c. is true. A sentence like: 'Mr Jameson needs drink' is likely to refer to alcohol (see **b**).

d. is not true. The aim is to *get* the specific gravity of his urine to that point so obviously it is not within that range at the moment.

e. is true. 'Out of the ordinary' means 'abnormal' or 'exceptional' or 'unusual'.

f. is not true. The Nursing Intervention recommends as much fruit as possible.

Exercise 12b

1 b

2 a

3 b

4 c

5 a 'To sit up' means to sit upright. 'To sit well up' is to sit even more upright.

6 a

Exercise 12c

Mr Jameson is taking in an <u>insufficient</u> quantity of fluid which is causing his skin <u>to become</u> dry. It is necessary to <u>ensure</u> the patient takes in <u>at least</u> 3000 ml of fluid every day and nurses must <u>sit</u> the patient upright before giving him an <u>hourly</u> drink.

The aim is to get Mr Jameson to produce more than 2000 ml of urine <u>every</u> day. It is <u>necessary</u> to measure the specific gravity of his urine. Any abnormalities out <u>of</u> the range of 1.010–1.025 <u>should</u> be reported.

Keep the patient's mouth, teeth and dentures <u>clean</u>. Ensure oral hygiene is done <u>every</u> four hours in order <u>to encourage</u> a flow of saliva to keep the patient's oropharyngeal muscles healthy.

Exercise 12d

a. You may get inaccurate results if/the urine is left exposed to the air/you leave the urine exposed to the air.

b. A healthy person's urine should not/have an unpleasant smell/smell unpleasant.

c. A smell like ammonia is/produced/made/by decomposing urine.

d. Sweet-smelling urine may indicate diabetes mellitus.

e. A urinary infection may be indicated by/urine that smells of fish/fish-smelling urine.

f. Dark-coloured urine indicates dehydration.

g. Specific gravity measures the concentration of substances dissolved in urine.

h. A range of 1.005 to 1.025 is normal for the specific gravity of urine.

i. A single measurement gives little information.

j. Diabetes insipidus or renal damage is indicated by low specific gravity.

Exercise 12e

How to get urine for testing

You should aim for a 'clean catch' urine sample which is <u>free from</u> contaminants. In the case of men, the head of the penis <u>should</u> be wiped clean. Women <u>should</u> first wash the area between the lips of the vulva with <u>soapy</u> water. <u>Use</u> a clean container and catch <u>between</u> 30–60 ml of urine after <u>allowing</u> the first small amount to fall into the toilet <u>bowl</u> so that you get your sample from <u>mid</u> stream.

Exercise 12f

1. The patient, Mr Robert Jameson, is becoming unco-operative.
2. He is refusing drinks that are offered to him and as a consequence his dehydration is getting worse.
3. He produced less than 1000 ml of dark-coloured urine on 16 September and the results of the test for specific gravity have dropped to a worrying 985.
4. Also he has had no bowel movement on 16 September.

Exercise 12g

A healthy human being will lose something like 2.4 litres of fluid every day in the form of sweat, urine, <u>exhaled</u> air and bowel movements. The feeling of thirst will normally <u>lag behind</u> the need to drink because it may take some time for your body <u>to pay attention</u> to the sensation of thirst.

If it is left too long, the body will start to show signs of dehydration such as feelings of <u>dizziness</u>. The body will become <u>flushed</u> and start sweating <u>profusely</u>. There is danger when the body actually *stops* sweating.

The best solution to dehydration is simply <u>to consume</u> plenty of water. Soft drinks manufacturers spend huge quantities of money on persuading us to buy their soft drink products but in fact the best choice is water. <u>Caffeinated</u> drinks as well as alcohol will in fact increase dehydration because they increase urine output.

Exercise 12h

a. These patients believe that no treatment will help them.
b. Telling medical staff that treatments have failed gives them satisfaction.
c. These patients are looking more for a long-term relationship with a medical practitioner than (for) relief from any illness.
d. Patients like these will often make practitioners feel guilty and inadequate.
e. Anyone who tries to help is defeated by these patients.
f. They get satisfaction only from their own self-destruction.
g. These patients should not be abandoned but worked with like patients with terminal cancer.

Exercise 12i

1 Extremely runny faeces is a characteristic of diarrhoea.

2 A patient with diarrhoea goes to the toilet a lot.

3 Runny stools are passed at least three times a day.

4 Passing large quantities of normal stools is not diarrhoea.

5 It is not the quantity but the degree of firmness that is important.

6 Diarrhoea is dangerous because it causes a rapid reduction of water and sodium which are both necessary for life.

7 Dehydration is often caused by continual diarrhoea that lasts fourteen days or more.

8 Early features of dehydration include dry mouth, thirst, weak pulse and when you pinch the skin it goes back slowly.

9 Oral rehydration therapy (ORT) does not stop the diarrhoea but it does put back lost fluids and essential salts.

10 Adding glucose to ORS solution enables the intestine to absorb fluid and salts more efficiently.

11 ORT is normally an adequate treatment for patients suffering from acute watery diarrhoea.

Exercise 12j

Fill in the spaces in the following passage about oral rehydration therapy with the correct word from the brackets.

You can use a simple salt/sugar solution for ORT. Mix a level teaspoon of salt with 8 level teaspoons of sugar in a litre of drinking water.

It is a good idea to use molasses or some other form of unrefined sugar because unrefined sugar contains more potassium than white sugar. Do not use too much salt because in some cases, salt can cause convulsions. Too little salt does no harm but it is less effective in preventing dehydration. As a rule of thumb for the amount of salt to use in the solution, it should taste no saltier than tears.

Chapter Thirteen

Mrs Pauline Dobson – dementia

Mrs Dobson is a psychogeriatric patient and has been in hospital for a long time. (She will eventually die there.) First, look at the list of some of the vocabulary which appears in this chapter. This is followed by an extract from the notes on Mrs Dobson's Patient Care Plan covering a period of three weeks.

VOCABULARY

to be a danger to oneself: to risk hurting oneself.

to settle: to become accustomed to a new situation.

agitated: upset, emotional.

distress: unhappiness.

tearful: crying a lot.

to lack emotional control: to have no control of feelings.

disorientated: unaware of where you are.

to supervise: to tell someone what to do.

overactive: too much manic energy.

to be apathetic: to have no interest in anything.

tangle: a confusing mix-up.

Date defined	Problems	Nursing intervention	Date resolved
8.2.01	Difficulty dressing & washing efficiently	1. Dressing programme – encourage patient to do as much as poss.	
8.2.01	Almost total absence of short-term memory	2. Constantly remind as to real situation	
8.2.01	Disorientation in time & place – e.g. sometimes thinks she is in her old place of work. Mistakes people around her for those she once knew	3. As with 2. Encourage to be sociable & join group activities. (Enjoys a Guinness)	
8.2.01	Rapid mood swings: behaviour ranges between: a. <u>overactive</u> (e.g. leaves ward to go home) & b. <u>apathetic</u> & drowsy (e.g. at times can barely walk)	4. Constant observation, tranquillisers as required Supervise adequate diet & fluids	
18.2.01	Broken & infected areas on: a. R ankle b. Neck c. Blister on R heel d. Lower parts of both legs	5. Daily saline bath Cover areas with dry Telfa dressings	23.2.01

Date defined	Problems	Nursing intervention	Date resolved
19.2.01	Dry mouth	6. At least one glass fluid with meals oral hygiene as required, in particular before meals	25.2.01
23.2.01	Fails to feed herself when in drowsy state	7. Needs feeding & encouragement	
28.2.01	Poor fluid intake	7. 200 ml hourly by mouth mouth care – 4-hourly Nurse per shift allocated to chat	
28.2.01	Chest infection	8. Antibiotics as prescribed TPR twice daily Suction as required	

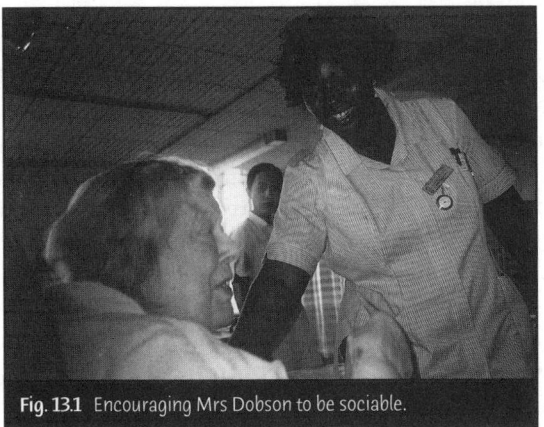

Fig. 13.1 Encouraging Mrs Dobson to be sociable.

Exercise 13a

From your reading of Mrs Dobson's Patient Care Plan notes, say which of the following statements are true:

1 On 8 February, Mrs Dobson was noted to:
a. be forgetful.
b. be forgotten.
c. recognise people from her past.
d. mismatch names with faces.
e. be aggressive.
f. be excited.
g. be excitable.
h. leave the hospital and go home.

2 On 8 February, nurses were instructed to:
a. dress the patient.
b. do as little as possible to help the patient dress.
c. remind Mrs Dobson of the time and place.
d. encourage the patient to party.

e. keep an eye on the patient.

f. regularly give the patient tranquillisers at regular intervals.

3 On 18 February, the patient had:

a. a saline bath.

b. an infected left foot.

c. a broken ankle.

d. infections on calves and shins.

4 Between 23 and 28 February, the patient:

a. deteriorated.

b. made some improvement.

c. was no longer able to feed herself.

d. sometimes wouldn't eat.

5 Between 23 and 28 February, nurses were instructed to:

a. brush Mrs Dobson's teeth four times an hour.

b. talk at the patient.

c. give regular suction.

d. take the patient's temperature every two days.

Exercise 13b

Mrs Dobson died in mid-March and her Patient Care Plan was used to write the following report after enquiries by relatives. As you read the report, fill in the gaps with words or phrases from the brackets:

Mrs Pauline Dobson was a patient in the psychogeriatric ward. By 18 September, it .... (was, is, will be) obvious that she .... (will be, was, is) suffering .... (with, by, from) serious memory loss. She couldn't remember things that .... (had, are, have) just happened.

She .... (have found, finds, found) it difficult to wash and dress herself and was often disoriented – she .... (will, may, would) forget where she .... (was, is, will be) and would get dates and times .... (mix, mixes, mixed) up.

Nursing staff .... (will be, are, were) encouraged to give her constant reminders of reality. They wanted her to be .... (as, by, with) self-sufficient as possible so Mrs Dobson .... (was, will be, is) encouraged to do as much for herself as she .... (could, can, will).

At this time the patient was suffering .... (from, by, of) mood swings. One minute she was 'high' and overactive and the .... (minute, next, later) she was lethargic and .... (sleep, sleepy, sleeping). During her low periods she .... (did, does, do) not have the energy to get up out of her chair. Tranquillisers .... (will be given, gave, were given) to help her .... (manage, handle, cope) with the manic periods.

On 18 February, nurses .... (identify, identified, identifying) infections .... (in, on, by) her neck legs and feet and the Staff Nurse recommended .... (every day, all day, daily) saline baths and for all infected areas to be .... (cover, covering, covered) with Telfa dressings.

On the following day, the patient complained ...... (of, with, by) a dry mouth and nursing staff .... (are, were, will be) instructed to give her mouthwashes .... (at, in, during) meal times and to .... (make, do, makes) sure that she .... (will drink, was drinking, were drinking) at least one glass of fluid with her meals.

By 23 February, Mrs Dobson's lethargic .... (condition, attitude, states) were noted to be getting .... (worse, bad, worst) and because she was unable to feed herself she .... (seemed to, appeared to, evidently) needed help at meal times.

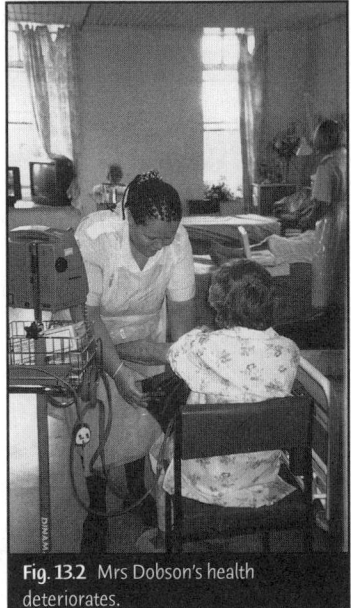

Fig. 13.2 Mrs Dobson's health deteriorates.

Five days .... (later, late, soon after) it was noted that Mrs Dobson was drinking very .... (small, not much, little) and the Staff Nurse recommended that staff keep Mrs Dobson .... (in, under, with) close watch. Nurses were .... (instructed, instruct, instructing) to see that she was .... (receiving, receive, received) at least 200 ml of fluid .... (all, total, every) hour to avoid ...... (dehydration, dehydrate, dehydrated). Because it was clear that Mrs Dobson was failing fast .... (the, a, some) nurse was allocated on .... (all, total, every) shift to spend some time sitting with her to keep her mind stimulated.

The patient .... (received, made, caught) a chest infection on 28 February and antibiotics .... (were, was, are) prescribed, TPR readings were taken twice daily and she ...... (is, were, was) given suction as and when necessary.

Exercise 13c

Put the following words into the spaces: **if, both, by, but, for, of, or, with, in. Some of them will be used more than once.**

Nursing guidelines for last offices

Ensure privacy .... the patient and relatives and inform .... the nursing office and portering staff. Remove all upper bedlinen .... leave a sheet to cover the patient.

Lay the patient flat, face up .... his limbs in a natural position and his arms .... his side.

Gently close the patient's eyelids.

Support the mandible .... a closed position with a light pillow and using a disposable bowl, manually express the bladder. Wash the patient and ...... the patient is male, shave him.

Remove all jewellery and list it .... the Patients' Valuables book .... the presence of two nurses.

Apply identification bands and cards .... the limbs and apply an incontinence pad .... disposable napkin.

Place the shroud .... position and wrap the body completely ....
the sheet which you should then secure with adhesive tape. Finally
inform the portering staff that the body is ready .... collection.

Exercise 13d

The following sentences describe the problem of dementia in greater detail. Rewrite each of the sentences so that they begin with the words underlined. The first one is done as an example:

Dementia has become a major problem in developed countries where the over-65s form a high percentage of the population. <u>The over 65s</u>

Answer: <u>The over 65s</u> form a high percentage of the population in developed countries and so dementia has become a major problem there.

1 In the UK there are 700 000 people with dementia and one-third of these are in hospitals. <u>Of the 700 000 people</u>

2 Dementia slowly destroys the brain cells. <u>The brain cells</u>

3 Scientists have described the physical characteristics as 'tangles' in the brain. <u>The physical characteristics</u>

4 Dementia causes a decline in the abilities to think, remember and learn. <u>The abilities to think,</u>

5 It becomes increasingly difficult, then finally impossible, to do simple things like washing, eating and dressing. <u>Simple things</u>

6 Some researchers say that dementia patients lose physical and mental abilities in exactly the reverse order that they acquired them when they were children. <u>Some researchers say that physical and mental abilities are lost</u>

7 Eventually a sufferer of Alzheimer's disease, the most common form of dementia, is able to smile but unable to speak or walk. <u>Eventually, though, a sufferer of Alzheimer's disease may</u>

Read the following article about the death of the well-known author Iris Murdoch.

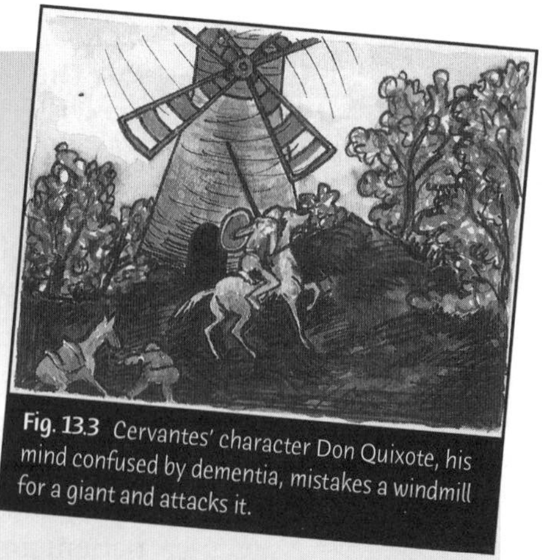

Fig. 13.3 Cervantes' character Don Quixote, his mind confused by dementia, mistakes a windmill for a giant and attacks it.

THE DEATH OF IRIS MURDOCH

Iris Murdoch, the award-winning writer from Ireland, died in February 1999 at the age of 79 after a long fight with Alzheimer's disease.

Before she died, she and her husband decided to donate her brain to research into the disease.

According to the Alzheimer's Disease Society, donations like this are essential in order to understand how the disease works. Professor Robin Jacoby who cared for Iris Murdoch in her final days said in a BBC interview 'researchers will use the brain to make microscope slides so that the lesions of Alzheimer's disease can be correlated with psychological defects that were found in life.'

Iris Murdoch herself described the disease in its early stages as 'a very very bad, quiet place'. Her husband who nursed her throughout her last years was with her when she died and after her death he wrote in his own book Iris: A Memoir, 'The voyage is over and under the dark escort of Alzheimer's she has arrived somewhere. So have I.'

Exercise 13e   **Which of the sentences out of a, b or c is grammatically correct?**

1   a. The decision to donate her brain was made jointly.
b. The decision to make a donation of her brain were made jointly.
c. The joint decision to donate her brain were made by Iris Murdoch and her husband.

2   a. A donated brain teach us about the disease.
b. Donated brains teach about the disease.
c. A donated brains teaches us about the disease.

3   a. Researchers can be able to match brain lesions with psychological problems.
b. It is possible for researchers to match lesions of the brain with psychological problems.
c. Researchers can be matching brain lesions by psychological problems.

4   a. Iris Murdoch's husband who was with her when she died.
b. With Iris Murdoch when she died were her husband.
c. When she died, Iris Murdoch's husband was there.

Exercise 13f   **These words are in the article 'The Death of Iris Murdoch'. Fit them into the spaces in the sentences that follow. Each one will need to be changed in some way:**

microscope

correlate

to die

donate

to understand

1   The ...... of Iris Murdoch was in 1999.

2   Researchers are always glad to receive ...... of organs.

3   The research is done at ...... level.

4   Researchers are looking for ...... between brain lesions and psychological defects.

5   Organ donations are essential for ...... of the disease.

Mr Jeffrey Topham died from cancer. It was the wish of both himself and his wife and children that he should die at home, so a nurse was allocated to help out. This is her account of the last few days of Mr Topham's life.

I first made it clear to Mrs Topham that we no longer have a cure in mind and that drugs would be administered only for the purposes of relieving pain and to enable Mr Topham to retain control of his bladder for as long as possible.

I suggested that we requisition a hospital bed in order to assist with bathing and giving the patient drinks but Mr Topham was quite insistent, saying that he wanted to die as naturally as possible in the same bed he had been born in.

He died on the Wednesday and in the days before he slipped in and out of a coma. I noticed that the skin around his feet and hands was cool. He drank little and so the fact that he was incontinent of both stools and urine did not matter much. His urine was a dark colour.

On Monday, Mr Topham was still conscious most of the time. He tried, at one point, to get out of bed and he fell to the floor. With Mrs Topham's help, I put a blanket under him and lifted him back on to the bed and very soon after this incident happened he began to slip in and out of a coma. I administered oxygen to help him breathe and gave atropine to dry up his throat a little. I showed Mrs Topham how to massage her husband's hands and back and how to use a folded sheet under his back to help with turning and lifting.

When I called on Tuesday, the patient was unconscious all of the time. His breathing became very irregular. Mrs Topham and I turned him every few hours. His chest rose and fell at irregular intervals sometimes with a pause of a minute or even longer. His eyes became glassy and finally by Wednesday morning there was no longer any breathing and no breath was coming from his nose. I called Dr Johnson and he pronounced him dead at ten o'clock that morning.

Exercise 13g   **Choose from a, b and c the best answer to the following questions:**

1 What does the nurse mean when she says 'we no longer had a cure in mind'?
a. We couldn't think of a cure.
b. We no longer thought of a cure.
c. We had decided not to cure him.

2 What does it mean to 'requisition a hospital bed'?
a. To buy a hospital bed.
b. To order a hospital bed.
c. To use a hospital bed.

3 The nurse says 'he slipped in and out of a coma'. What does this mean?
a. To be conscious sometimes.
b. To have accidents when unconscious.
c. To be unconscious all the time.

4 What happened on Tuesday?
a. Mr Topham was breathing steadily.
b. Mr Topham's breathing was unsteady.
c. Mr Topham's breathing steadied.

5 The nurse says 'his eyes became glassy'. What does this mean?
a. His eyes were dull.
b. He was given his glasses to wear.
c. His eyes were shiny.

Exercise 13h   **The following words are taken from the text above. Adapt them and put them into the spaces in these sentences.**

irregular

interval

bladder control

coma

cool

happened

naturally

relief

slip

1 Chemotherapy or radiation is sometimes given to .... pain of a dying person. (Meaning: to ease)

2 Dying patients may well experience pain caused by a growing tumour or be unable to use their legs or lose .... (Meaning: become incontinent)

3 Medical treatment during the final days aims to keep dying patients comfortable and allow them to have a .... death. (Meaning: without too much chemical assistance)

4 When someone has advanced cancer, dying often occurs slowly. Each day the patient grows weaker and weaker and will often .... in and out of consciousness. (Meaning: to move from one state to another without much effort)

5 Near the end of life you can expect a patient to breathe .... (Meaning: not in a uniform way)

6 Sometimes there will be long ...... between breaths. (Meaning: pauses)

7 Sometimes a person who is .... may suddenly open their eyes. This may surprise you – they don't usually talk but are awake for some time. (Meaning: in a coma)

8 The skin will be .... than normal and it will be a different colour – usually blue grey. (Meaning: not warm, but not cold)

9 It is not always clear when death .... but it is normally a moment of intense silence and stillness. (Meaning: takes place/occurs)

Elderly people in the UK today

VOCABULARY

celibate: not having sex.

well into: a long way into.

correlation: relationship/connection.

in isolation: alone and with no contact with others.

mobility: the ability to move around (be mobile).

pensioner: a retired person who is receiving a pension.

deprivation: not having enough food, warmth, etc.

Research by old age charities has identified that a combination of sex and money is the key to a long life.

The research shows that sexually active older people live longer and stay healthier than people who are celibate. The research shows that women in particular remain interested in sex well into old age and that elderly people who are sexually active are healthier.

There is a definite correlation between wealth and health and people who live in isolation die earlier than those who live with a partner and have grandchildren to keep them company. Old people, who feel they have lived (and continue to live) active and useful lives, regardless of religious beliefs, say they do not fear death.

However, isolation and poverty are still major problems in the UK and have a major impact on the health of elderly people. Isolation is related to mobility and so public transport plays a major role in their lives. The ability to move freely around is linked with a sense of general well-being and this is good for health. The argument is that if life were better, there would be less spent on healthcare.

The research also shows that two-thirds of pensioners in the UK live at some level of deprivation and that 45% of them live in poverty. In fact 15% of the pensioners who were interviewed for the research said that at some time they had gone without food.

Exercise 13i

The following sentences are taken from the text you have just read. Re-write these sentences so that your re-written sentences begin with the words in brackets.

The first is done for you as an example.

a. A combination of sex and money is the key to a long life. (Sex and money combined...)

Answer: Sex and money combined is the key to a long life.

b. Sexually active older people live longer and stay healthier than people who are celibate. (The lives of sexually active people are ......)

c. Some old people say they do not fear death. ('We do not ......)

d. Elderly people who are sexually active are healthier. (If elderly people ......)

e. People who live in isolation die earlier (People whose lives ......)

Exercise 13j

Complete the short text that follows by filling in the spaces.

There is a clear correlation .... health and .... sense .... well-being. As well-being is linked .... sexuality and money so celibacy and poverty are related .... ill-health and a short life. The two-thirds .... the population that live in poverty die earlier .... those who live fulfilled lives.

Exercise 13k

Read the following two sentences:

Dementia affects 0–5% of those aged 60–70, 20% of those over 80 and 30% of people aged 90+. Over the age of 65, one in 100 have Parkinson's disease.

The sentences are re-written below with exactly the same information. Fill in the spaces with a suitable word:

Dementia affects ...... 0 ...... 5% of those aged ...... 60 ...... 70, 20% of those who are 80 and ...... and 30% of people aged 90 or ...... Out of ...... 100 people aged 65 or ......, one .... Parkinson's disease.

Exercise 13l: Further practice

Read these notes and fill in the form that follows:

Gurdip Singh is 87. He was admitted unconscious (scoring 6 on the Glasgow Coma Scale) after a serious fall in which he injured his head. Two weeks later, he is still unconscious and he is totally dependant for all personal cleansing and it is necessary to look out for pressure sores and to keep his skin clean and his hair untangled. There is also a potential problem of dehydration and weight loss. He is normally 70 kg and he should be kept at this weight if possible. There is a risk of dehydration and it is important to maintain the patient's intake of fluids and keep defecation and urination to patient's normal frequency.

Problems	Goals
Problem 1	
Problem 2	
Problem 3	

Answers and comments on the language

Exercise 13a

1   a. is true. However, the word 'forgetful' is a rather inaccurate way to describe Mrs Dobson. 'Forgetful' really describes someone who forgets things rather than someone who seems to have forgotten almost everything.
b. is not true.
c. is not true. She is remembering people from the past but mixing them up with people in the present.
d. is true. To 'mismatch' is to put the wrong things together. People can be 'mismatched'. So for example can sheets be mismatched with beds.
e. is not true.
f. is not true. 'Excited' would normally mean she is looking forward to something and feeling happy.
g. is true. 'Excitable' describes an emotionally 'high' state or someone who gets 'high' easily. It can mean angry and aggressive and nearly out of control.

h. is not true. In the notes (18/2/01) it says 'leaves ward to go home' which means that she intended to go home, she didn't actually go. If she had gone home the notes would say 'left ward and went home.'

2   a. is not true.

b. is true. The instructions to 'encourage patient to do as much as possible' suggest that nurses should do as little as possible for her so that Mrs Dobson has to do as much as possible for herself.

c. is true. The instructions to 'constantly remind as to real situation' mean bringing Mrs Dobson's attention to the 'here and now'.

d. is not true. 'Group activities' might include a party but really suggest things like Bingo and TV.

e. is true. The expression in the notes 'constant observation' means 'keep an eye on…' or 'be vigilant over…'.

f. is not true. 'Tranquillisers as required' means given at irregular intervals – as and when they are needed.

3   a. is true.

b. is not true.

c. is not true. Broken skin but no broken bones.

d. is true. Note vocabulary: 'calves' (singular 'calf') – back part of the lower leg. 'Shin' – front part of the lower leg.

4   a. is true. At this point the patient was going downhill fast.

b. is true. You will see that the problems with her feet and legs noted on 18/2/01 were 'resolved' by 23/2/01. 'Some' improvement is 'a little' improvement.

c. is true. She was unable to feed herself when in a 'low' period.

d. is not true. 'She wouldn't eat' here suggests that she *refused* to eat, whereas at times Mrs Dobson forgot to eat.

5   a. is not true. '4-hourly' means every 4 hours.

b. is not true. The preposition that goes with 'talk' is important. 'To talk at' means to lecture someone – or at least to talk so that they don't get a chance to reply. 'To talk with' and 'to talk to' mean to have a two-way conversation.

c. is not true. Suction should be given 'as required'. 'Regular suction' is really suction at set times. However, people sometimes use it to mean 'often'.

d. is not true. 'TPR twice daily' means two TPRs every day.

Exercise 13b

Mrs Pauline Dobson was a patient in the psychogeriatric ward. By 18 September, it <u>was</u> obvious that she <u>was</u> suffering from serious memory loss. She couldn't remember things that <u>had</u> just happened.

She <u>found</u> it difficult to wash and dress herself and was often disoriented – she <u>would</u> forget where she <u>was</u> and would get dates and times <u>mixed</u> up.

Nursing staff <u>were</u> encouraged to give her constant reminders of reality. They wanted her to be <u>as</u> self-sufficient as possible so Mrs Dobson <u>was</u> encouraged to do as much for herself as she <u>could</u>.

At this time the patient was suffering <u>from</u> mood swings. One minute she was 'high' and overactive and the <u>next</u> she was lethargic and <u>sleepy</u>. During her low periods she <u>did</u> not have the energy to get up out of her chair. Tranquillisers <u>were given</u> to help her <u>cope</u> with the manic periods.

On 18 February, nurses <u>identified</u> infections <u>on</u> her neck, legs and feet and the Staff Nurse recommended <u>daily</u> saline baths and for all infected areas to be <u>covered</u> with Telfa dressings.

On the following day, the patient complained <u>of</u> a dry mouth and nursing staff <u>were</u> instructed to give her mouthwashes <u>at</u> meal times and to <u>make</u> sure that she <u>was drinking</u> at least one glass of fluid with her meals.

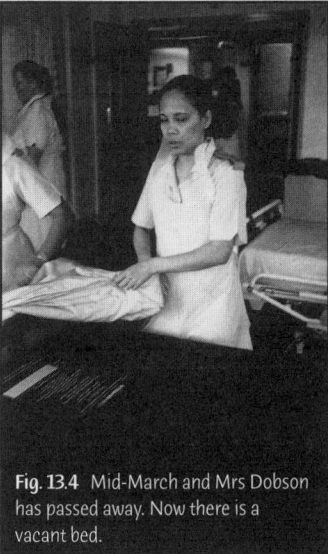

Fig. 13.4 Mid-March and Mrs Dobson has passed away. Now there is a vacant bed.

By 23 February, Mrs Dobson's lethargic <u>states</u> were noted to be getting <u>worse</u> and because she was unable to feed herself she <u>evidently</u> needed help at meal times.

Five days <u>later</u> it was noted that Mrs Dobson was drinking very <u>little</u> and the Staff Nurse recommended that staff keep Mrs Dobson <u>under</u> close watch. Nurses were <u>instructed</u> to see that she was <u>receiving</u> at least 200 ml of fluid <u>every</u> hour to avoid <u>dehydration</u>. Because it was clear that Mrs Dobson was failing fast <u>a</u> nurse was allocated on <u>every</u> shift to spend some time sitting with her to keep her mind stimulated.

The patient <u>caught</u> a chest infection on 28 February and antibiotics <u>were</u> prescribed, TPR readings were taken twice daily and she <u>was</u> given suction as and when necessary.

Exercise 13c

Nursing guidelines for last offices

Ensure privacy <u>for</u> the patient and relatives and inform <u>both</u> the nursing office and portering staff. Remove all upper bedlinen <u>but</u> leave a sheet to cover the patient.

Lay the patient flat, face up <u>with</u> his limbs in a natural position and his arms <u>by</u> his side.

Gently close the patient's eyelids.

Support the mandible <u>in</u> a closed position with a light pillow and using a disposable bowl, manually express the bladder. Wash the patient and <u>if</u> the patient is male, shave him.

Remove all jewellery and list it <u>in</u> the Patients' Valuables book <u>in</u> the presence of two nurses.

Apply identification bands and cards <u>to</u> the limbs and apply an incontinence pad <u>or</u> disposable napkin.

Place the shroud <u>in</u> position and wrap the body completely <u>in</u> <u>with</u> the sheet which you should then secure with adhesive tape. Finally inform the portering staff that the body is ready <u>for</u> collection.

Exercise 13d

1 Of the 70 000 people in the UK with dementia, one-third are in hospitals.

2 The brain cells are slowly destroyed by dementia.

3 The physical characteristics have been described by scientists as 'tangles' in the brain.

4 The abilities to think, remember and learn decline because of dementia.

5 Simple things like washing, eating and drinking become difficult then finally impossible to do.

6 Some researchers say that physical and mental abilities are lost by dementia patients in exactly the reverse order that they acquired them when they were children.

7 Eventually, though a sufferer of Alzheimer's disease may be able to smile, he is unable to speak or walk.

Exercise 13e

1 a.

2 b.

3 b.

4 c.

Exercise 13f

1 The <u>death</u> of Iris Murdoch was in 1999.

2 Researchers are always glad to receive <u>donations</u> of organs.

3 The research is done at <u>microscopic</u> level.

4 Researchers are looking for <u>correlations</u> between brain lesions and psychological defects.

5 Organ donations are essential for <u>an understanding</u> of disease.

Exercise 13g

1 **b.** To have something 'in mind' is to be thinking about it and planning for it. Option **a** suggests that there is a cure but we don't know what it is.

2 **b.** Hospital wards often 'requisition' things like equipment, furniture and other materials. There are requisition forms and documents for doing so. When things like equipment are kept in a store they are 'requisitioned' for use as and when they are needed.

3 **a.** The verb to 'slip' has many uses. For example, people talk about 'slipping on' a pair of shoes. Soap is 'slippery', baths have 'slip mats' and so on. Usually 'slip' suggests a minimum of effort involved so 'to slip in and out of consciousness' means 'to become unconscious easily'.

4 **b.** 'Unsteady' means 'not regular and rather weak'. A sick person might be described as 'unsteady on their feet'. To 'steady' (option **c**) means 'to become regular'.

5 **a.** You would expect 'glassy' to mean shiny and bright like glass but the opposite is true when used about eyes. 'The water was glassy' means that the water was perfectly still.

Exercise 13h

1 Chemotherapy or radiation is sometimes given to <u>relieve</u> pain of a dying person.

2 Dying patients may well experience pain caused by a growing tumour or be unable to use their legs or lose <u>bladder control</u>.

3 Medical treatment during the final days aims to keep dying patients comfortable and allow them to have a <u>natural</u> death.

4 When someone has advanced cancer, dying often occurs slowly. Each day the patient grows weaker and weaker and will often <u>slip</u> in and out of consciousness.

5 Near the end of life you can expect a patient to breathe <u>irregularly</u>.

6 Sometimes there will be long <u>intervals</u> between breaths.

7 Sometimes a person who is <u>comatosed</u> may suddenly open their eyes. This may surprise you – they don't usually talk but are awake for some time.

8 The skin will be <u>cooler</u> than normal and it will be a different colour – usually blue-grey.

9 It is not always clear when death <u>happens</u> but it is normally a moment of intense silence and stillness.

Exercise 13i

b. The lives of sexually active people are longer and healthier than the lives of people who are celibate.
c. 'We do not fear death' some old people say.
d. If elderly people are sexually active they are healthier.
e. People whose lives are isolated die earlier.

Exercise 13j

There is a clear correlation <u>between</u> health and <u>a</u> sense <u>of</u> well-being. As well-being is linked <u>to/with</u> sexuality and money so celibacy and poverty are related <u>to</u> ill-health and a short life. The two-thirds <u>of</u> the population that live in poverty die earlier <u>than</u> those who live fulfilled lives.

Exercise 13k

Dementia affects <u>between</u> 0 <u>and</u> 5% of those aged <u>between</u> 60 <u>and</u> 70, 20% of those who are 80 and <u>over</u> and 30% of people aged 90 or <u>more</u>. Out of <u>every</u> 100 people aged 65 or <u>over/more</u>, one <u>has</u> Parkinson's disease.

Exercise 13l: Further practice

Problems	Goals
Problem 1 Danger of pressure sores	Keep skin & hair groomed and clean.
Problem 2 Risk of dehydration	Maintain hydration Return defecation & urination to normal.
Problem 3 Risk of weight loss	Maintain weight at 70 kg.

Chapter Fourteen

Discharge from hospital

Miss Anne Barton is being discharged from hospital to a care home. Look at the vocabulary list first then study Miss Barton's Discharge Summary that follows.

DISCHARGE SUMMARY

Patient
Miss Anne Barton

Age 82 years

D.O.B. 2 Aug 1918

Date of Discharge
June 10, 2000

Date of Admission
March 5, 2000

PROBLEMS

1. Multiple CVAs with bilateral hemiplegia. Needs max. assistance with ADLs and mobility – 2 people to assist with movement. Dressing, washing and bathing done by staff.
2. Continent of urine if routinely toileted during the day – occasionally incontinent of urine at night.
3. Prone to constipation – has soft-formed stools when toileted – needs occasional glycerine suppository. Receives Metamucil 15 ml daily.
4. Essential hypertension – BP ranges from 150/90 to 184/108 – monitored 2 days per week (Tues. and Fri.).
5. History of depression – withdrawn and weepy at times. Minimal response to antidepressant drugs (amitriptyline 25 mg – was D/C May 1998). Family has visited frequently and v. supportive.
6. Progressive dysphasia – speech slurred – difficult to understand. V. slow to respond. Thanks staff for help.

Next of kin
Ray Barton
phone 0123 434 908 (brother)

Sue Brown
phone 0987 610 896 (niece)

Medical regimen
Metamucil 15 ml daily.
Nadolol 80 g daily.
Brandy 30 cc daily.

Safety needs
Vision – good/able to read clock on the wall and small print.
Hearing – can hear normal conversation.
Mechanical aids – side-rails and support in chair with pillows and belt restraints.
Trunk balance poor.
Well oriented to time/place/person.

Strengths and resources
Gets help from family. Concerned about appearance and feels comfortable letting staff know what her needs are. Wants to move to a geriatric facility in York as it is much closer for family to visit – family visits 2–3 × weekly.

VOCABULARY

weepy: cries, unhappy, tearful.

slurred: one word seems to run into another.

oriented: aware of things around you and able to deal with them.

trunk: abdomen – from waist to shoulders.

progressive: worsening.

continent: can control toileting.

restraints: belts to hold someone in place.

to toilet: to take (someone) to the toilet or make sure they go to the toilet.

geriatric facility: old people's care home.

Exercise 14a

Which of the following statements are correct?

a. Miss Barton has a stroke.
b. Miss Barton has had a stroke.
c. She can do most things for herself.
d. Miss Barton cannot control her bladder.
e. Miss Barton very rarely has constipation.
f. The patient's blood pressure is higher than normal.
g. The patient is alone in the world.
h. Amitriptyline makes little difference.
i. Her dysphasia is getting worse.
j. The patient doesn't know where she is.
k. Miss Barton has lost interest in what she looks like.

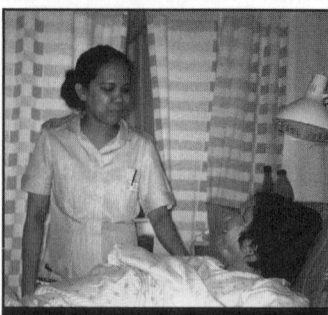

Fig. 14.1 Later the nurse writes in the notes that Miss Barton is 'well oriented to time, place and person.'

Exercise 14b

The following are extracts from Miss Barton's Discharge Summary. They are in their original note form. Add words to the brackets to turn the notes into 'full' sentences. The first is done as an example:

(   ) continent of urine if (   ) routinely toileted during the day.

Answer: **(She is)** continent of urine if **(she is)** routinely toileted during the day.

a. Dressing, washing and bathing (   ) done by staff.
b. (   ) history of depression. (   ) withdrawn and weepy at times.
c. (   ) progressive dysphasia (   ) speech (   ) slurred (   ) difficult to understand.
d. (   ) very slow to respond (   ) thanks staff for (   ) help.
e. (   ) trunk balance (   ) poor.

Exercise 14c

Miss Barton is 'continent of urine if toileted during the day'. This suggests that she is 'incontinent of urine if untoileted during the day.'

The negative version of continent is *in*continent and the negative version of toileted is *un*toileted.

Make negative versions of the following words using either un-, in-, non-, or dis-. (In some cases there is more than one possible answer.)

a. progressive.
b. prone.
c. routine.
d. assisted.
e. responsive.
f. restrained.
g. oriented.
h. concerned.
i. frequent.
j. support.

Exercise 14d

Rewrite the following sentences by using the negative forms of the words in Exercise 14c. (The first is done as an example):

The patient needs help when dressing herself.

Answer: the patient can dress herself <u>unassisted.</u>

a. She will not answer when spoken to.
b. The patient's family does not help her.
c. The patient is not aware of time and place.
d. We are not worried about her condition.
e. The patient does not urinate often.

Exercise 14e

The following is information about Miss Barton's medical problems. Fill in the gaps in the text using one word from each of the brackets:

Miss Barton .... (suffering with, suffers from, is suffering) essential hypertension and her blood pressure .... (range to, range from, ranges from) 150/90 to 184/108 mmHg. Her essential hypertension .... (might be due, may be because, might be caused) to a narrowing of the arteries, more blood .... (as, like, than) normal or the heart beating faster than it should.

If another medical problem such as kidney disease .... (will cause, causes, was causing) her high blood pressure, then her condition would be called 'secondary' hypertension.

Blood pressure is recorded in two values, e.g. 120/80 mmHg. The first or systolic value is ...... (a, the, some) pressure of the blood .... (with an artery wall, against the artery walls, by the artery wall) when the heart contracts. The second or diastolic value is .... (a, the, some) pressure against the artery walls when the heart relaxes .... (after beating, when beating, between beats). A desirable blood pressure for healthy adults is 120/80 mmHg. Any blood pressure like Miss Barton's that .... (would stay, stays, stayed) at 140/90 mmHg or higher is .... (considerably, considered, considerable) high.

Miss Barton has .... (dysphasic, a dysphasia, dysphasia) as a result of a stroke so she finds it difficult .... (communication, to communicate, communicate) with others. People who have contact with her may need some .... (guidance, guide, guided) about how to talk with her. For example, they may need .... (remind, reminder, to be reminded) that she has not become .... (less, not, under) intelligent simply because she finds speaking difficult.

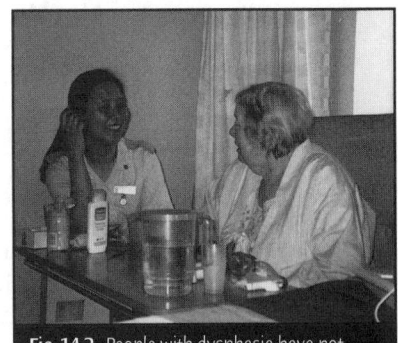

Fig. 14.2 People with dysphasia have not suddenly become less intelligent. They just find speaking difficult.

People talking with .... (dysphasia, a dysphasic, dysphasic) patients are advised not to ...... (rushing, rushed, rush) things, nor .... (interruption, interrupt, interrupted) patients when they are trying to talk and .... (need, have, should) try to use short sentences and short words. Writing things down and .... (use, using, used) drawings can help. Above all, they should not .... (get, have, are) discouraged if communication seems completely impossible.

Exercise 14f

Put these words into the gaps in this text about Miss Barton's discharge. as, with, to, by, for, who, from, at, in, of

For Miss Barton, discharge .... hospital could be a critical stage .... her life. The skills she acquired .... hospital .... regards eating, washing and dressing may be difficult .... transfer .... the new environment of the geriatric facility .... York that she is going .... Furthermore, elderly people like Miss Barton .... take drugs .... depression are often misdiagnosed and treated .... dementia when ...... fact symptoms .... confusion, memory loss, disorientation, increased anxiety and rapid breathing may be produced .... the drugs which are used .... treat her depression.

In the UK, elderly people like Miss Barton account .... 18% of the population but they consume 45% .... all prescription drugs and a recent study has shown that 97% ...... elderly people ...... nursing homes were taking prescription drugs compared with 71% ...... those living in the community.

People living .... nursing homes are therefore most .... risk .... misdiagnosis and it is important .... patients like Miss Barton .... be aware that symptoms that look like dementia could be something else.

Exercise 14g

Now read the following information about Mrs Martha Collins, who is also being discharged. As you read, fill in the gaps in the text.

Mrs Martha Collins ...... (is, was, are) 80 years old. She was .... (birth, born, given birth) on 17 September 1921. She ...... (had, has had, had) a history of hypertension and degenerative joint disease.

She ...... (had, has, had had) a fall on 13 April and .... (will be, were, was) immediately admitted to hospital. She has complained that she needs to frequently .... (go, going, go to) the toilet.

She was diagnosed with a left pneumonia and a urinary tract infection. Both .... (are treated, were treated, will be treated) with antibiotics during her hospitalisation. She also received physiotherapy to help her adjust .... (on, to, by) a walker (walking aid).

Mrs Collins lives in sheltered accommodation .... (where, who, which) help is provided for the residents with shopping, cleaning and house maintenance. Mrs Collins .... (have, has, is) no family. The bathroom in her flat is not .... (given, fixed, equipped) with a bath seat or safety rails and the patient needs some assistance with ....

(bathing and dressing, bath and dress, bathed and dressed). She can cook her own meals.

Mrs Collins needs to .... (visit, visited, be visited) by a nurse twice a week to monitor medications. She will also require home help 5 times a week .... (for, at, by) 4–6 hours a day to .... (assisting, assisted, assist) bathing and dressing. She needs to .... (use, get, make) physiotherapy 3 times a week to help her walking.

Exercise 14h Use the information in Exercise 14g to complete Mrs Collins' Discharge Summary. Fill in the gaps by choosing either a, b or c from the options provided.

DISCHARGE SUMMARY

Patient Mrs Martha Collins   **D.O.B.** 17/9/21

Date of Discharge 30 May 2001   **Date of Admission** 13 April 2001

PROBLEMS

1 Either: a. Used to suffer from hypertension and degenerative bone disease.
   Or: b. Has been suffering from hypertension & degenerative bone disease.
   Or: c. Will suffer from hypertension and degenerative bone disease.

2 Either: a. Needs to urinate frequently.
   Or: b. Produces a lot of urine.
   Or: c. Irregular urine.

3 Diagnosed – left pneumonia & urinary tract infection.

4 Needs assistance with walking/dressing/washing.

5 Either: a. Cannot use a walker.
   Or: b. Needs an adjustable walker.
   Or: c. Finds walker difficult.

Next of kin
No immediate family.

Needs
1. Bath seat and safety rails in bathroom.

2. Either: a. Nurse to visit every 2 weeks to monitor medications.
   Or: b. Nurse to visit 2 × week to monitor medications.
   Or: c. Visit a nurse 2 × week to monitor medications.

3 Either: a. Home help for 5 weeks.
   Or: b. Home help 5 × week 4-6 h.
   Or: c. 5 Home helps every week 4-6 h.

4 Physiotherapy 3 × week.

Strengths and resources
Independent-minded woman, fully alert and articulate, can cook.

Exercise 14i Just before Mrs Collins was discharged from hospital a nurse was asked to complete the following questionnaire about her to pass on to Mrs Collins' Community Nurse. Fill in the questionnaire using the information you have read about Mrs Collins:

QUESTIONNAIRE

Name	DOB	Discharge date
Mrs Martha Collins	17/9/21	30/5/03

Please read the following statements and tick appropriate boxes.

	Always/ totally	Often/ a lot	Sometimes /a little	Never/ nothing
Patient needs help dressing.				
Patient needs help to use the toilet.				
Patient needs a nurse in attendance at home.				
Patient needs help with making meals.				
Patient needs medications monitoring.				
Patient needs help with bathing.				
Patient needs mechanical aid to walk.				
Patient needs physiotherapy.				

Exercise 14i: Further practice

Read the following notes and complete the section of the Discharge Summary that follows:

Mr Peter Lawson was 79 when he was admitted to hospital after a fall in his bathroom at home. After four days of observation, he was discharged. His wife had died two months previously. This hit Mr Lawson hard and he values any chance to talk about her and their life together. He had never cooked until his wife's death and has been living on sandwiches and canned soup. He says he has always been constipated and takes two Beecham's pills every night. It would be best to change this habit and encourage Mr Lawson to have a bran-rich diet to achieve daily bowel movements.

Since his fall he has lost confidence in using the bath, even though his bath does have a slip mat. A neighbour cuts his hair and does his washing and Mr Lawson, whose vision and hearing are quite good, can walk unaided into the local village to do shopping.

Social Services have been involved in the case but it is necessary to confirm that Meals on Wheels will be provided daily and grab-rails installed at the side of his bath.

DISCHARGE SUMMARY

Problems

Needs

Strengths and resources

Answers and comments on the language

Exercise 14a

a. is incorrect. The stroke is an event in the past even though the effects of it exist in the present.

b. is correct. This is the correct tense and it tells us that the stroke happened in the recent past and Miss Barton is still suffering from the effects of it.

c. is incorrect. She 'needs 2 people to assist (her) with movement and ADLs' (Activities of Daily Living).

d. is incorrect. She is described as 'continent of urine'.

e. is incorrect. She is 'prone to constipation'. This means she 'tends to get constipation' or 'becomes constipated easily'.

f. is correct. Her blood pressure ranges from 150/90 to 184/108.

g. is incorrect. Miss Barton's family is 'v. (very) supportive'.

h. is correct. 'Amitriptyline was D/C in May' (discontinued/stopped).

i. is correct. Her dysphasia is described as 'progressive'.

j. is incorrect. She is 'well oriented to time/place/person'. This means she is aware of reality: when, where and who.

k. is incorrect. She is 'concerned' about her appearance. 'Concerned' here does not mean 'worried' but 'interested in' or 'cares about'.

Exercise 14b

a. Dressing, washing and bathing (are) done by staff.

b. (She has a) history of depression. (She is) withdrawn and weepy at times.

c. (She has) progressive dysphasia (and her) speech (is) slurred (and) difficult to understand.

d. (She is) very slow to respond (but) thanks staff for (their) help.

e. (Her) trunk balance (is) poor.

Exercise 14c

a. non-progressive.

b. non-prone.

c. non-routine.

d. unassisted.

e. unresponsive. (Sometimes non-responsive)

f. unrestrained. (Sometimes non-restrained)

g. disoriented.

h. unconcerned.

i. infrequent.

j. unsupportive.

Exercise 14d

a. She is unresponsive.

b. The patient's family is unsupportive.

c. The patient is disoriented.

d. We are unconcerned about her condition.

e. The patient urinates infrequently.

Exercise 14e

Miss Barton <u>suffers from</u> essential hypertension and her blood pressure <u>ranges from</u> 150/90 to 184/108. Her essential hypertension <u>might be due</u> to a narrowing of the arteries, more blood <u>than</u> normal or the heart beating faster than it should.

If another medical problem such as kidney disease <u>was causing</u> her high blood pressure, then her condition would be called 'secondary' hypertension.

Blood pressure is recorded in two values, e.g. 120/80 mmHg. The first or systolic is <u>the</u> pressure of the blood <u>against the artery walls</u> when the heart contracts. The second or diastolic value is <u>the</u> pressure against the artery walls when the heart relaxes <u>between beats</u>. A desirable blood pressure for healthy adults is 120/80 mmHg. Any blood pressure like Miss Barton's that <u>stays</u> at 140/90 mmHg or higher is <u>considered</u> high.

Miss Barton has <u>dysphasia</u> as a result of a stroke so she finds it difficult <u>to</u> <u>communicate</u> with others. People who have contact with her may need some <u>guidance</u> about how to talk with her. For example, they may need <u>to be reminded</u> that she has not become <u>less</u> intelligent simply because she finds speaking difficult.

People talking with <u>dysphasic</u> patients are advised not to <u>rush</u> things, nor <u>interrupt</u> patients when they are trying to talk and <u>should</u> try to use short sentences and short words. Writing things down and <u>using</u> drawings can help. Above all, they should not <u>get</u> discouraged if communication seems completely impossible.

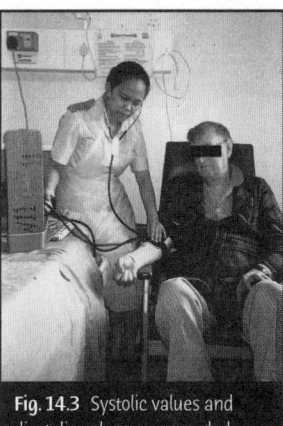

Fig. 14.3 Systolic values and diastolic values are recorded.

Exercise 14f

For Miss Barton, discharge <u>from</u> hospital could be a critical stage <u>in</u> her life. The skills she acquired <u>in</u> hospital <u>as</u> regards eating, washing and dressing may be difficult <u>to</u> transfer <u>to</u> the new environment of the geriatric facility <u>in</u> York that she is going <u>to</u>. Furthermore, elderly people like Miss Barton <u>who</u> take drugs <u>for</u> depression are often misdiagnosed and treated <u>for</u> dementia when <u>in</u> fact symptoms <u>of</u> confusion, memory loss, disorientation, increased anxiety and rapid breathing may be produced <u>by</u> the drugs which are used <u>to</u> treat her depression.

In the UK, elderly people like Miss Barton account <u>for</u> 18% of the population but they consume 45% <u>of</u> all prescription drugs and a recent study has shown that 97% <u>of</u> elderly people <u>in</u> nursing homes were taking prescription drugs compared with 71% <u>of</u> those living in the community.

People living <u>in</u> nursing homes are therefore most <u>at</u> risk <u>of</u> misdiagnosis and it is important <u>with</u> patients like Miss Barton <u>to</u> be aware that symptoms that look like dementia could be something else.

Exercise 14g

Mrs Martha Collins <u>is</u> 80 years old. She was <u>born</u> on 17 September 1921. She <u>has had</u> a history of hypertension and degenerative joint disease.

She <u>had</u> a fall on 13 April and <u>was</u> immediately admitted to hospital. She has complained that she needs to frequently <u>go</u> <u>to</u> the toilet.

She was diagnosed with a left pneumonia and a urinary tract infection. Both <u>were treated</u> with antibiotics during her hospitalisation. She also received physiotherapy to help her adjust <u>to</u> a walker (walking aid).

Mrs Collins lives in sheltered accommodation <u>where</u> help is provided for the residents with shopping, cleaning and house maintenance. Mrs Collins <u>has</u> no family. The bathroom in her flat is not <u>equipped</u> with a bath seat or safety rails and the patient needs some assistance with <u>bathing and dressing</u>. She can cook her own meals.

Mrs Collins needs to <u>be visited</u> by a nurse twice a week to monitor medications. She will also require home help 5 times a week <u>for</u> 4–6 hours a day to <u>assist</u> bathing and dressing. She needs to <u>get</u> physiotherapy 3 times a week to help her walking.

Exercise 14h

DISCHARGE SUMMARY

Problems

1. **b.** Has been suffering from hypertension & degenerative bone disease. Option **a** means that she did suffer once but now no longer does.
2. **a.** Needs to urinate frequently.
5. **c.** Finds walker difficult. The text tells us that she needed to 'adjust to a walker'.

Needs

2. **b.** Nurse to visit 2 × week to monitor medications.
3. **b.** Home help 5 × week 4–6 h.

Exercise 14i

QUESTIONNAIRE

Name	DOB	Discharge date
Mrs Martha Collins	17/9/21	30/5/01

Please read the following statements and tick appropriate boxes.

	Always/ totally	Often/ a lot	Sometimes /a little	Never/ nothing
Patient needs help dressing.		✓		
Patient needs help to use the toilet.		✓		
Patient needs a nurse in attendance at home.			✓	
Patient needs help with making meals.				✓
Patient needs medications monitoring.			✓	
Patient needs help with bathing.		✓		
Patient needs mechanical aid to walk.	✓			
Patient needs physiotherapy.		✓		

Exercise 14i: Further practice

DISCHARGE SUMMARY

Problems

1. grieving over loss of wife (died 2 months ago).
2. cannot cook.
3. constipated.
4. afraid of falling again whilst using bath.

Needs

1. to talk about wife.
2. daily Meals on Wheels.
3. bran-rich diet – move bowels daily.
4. grab-rails in bathroom.

Strengths and resources

1. help from neighbour with washing, etc.
2. vision and hearing reasonable.
3. mobile enough to walk to village shops.

Chapter Fifteen

Mr Albert Jones – HIV and drug abuse

Albert Jones has human immunodeficiency virus (HIV). This is his story in his own words:

> I started doing drugs back in the 1980s when I got into the punk rock scene – you know, drinking, acid and that. This led to coke then brown. So by the time I was 21 I was addicted and no longer into music.
>
> I was an addict but I was responsible when it came to works. I lived with these friends who told me that if I didn't quit they'd kick me out. 'OK', I said and agreed to go to rehab. and so I threw out my points. But like, there was no space at the rehab. clinic and they put me on the waiting list. I went back to the pad, got sick and then it dawned on me that I had thrown out my works. I scrambled but I got a point from a girl I hardly knew. That was my only time sharing but it only takes once. Funny though, it was the best hit I ever had. The clinic told me I was HIV in 1998.

Exercise 15a	A lot of what Albert Jones says is colloquial and may be difficult to understand. Some of the vocabulary he uses is given below. Work out what he means by choosing the nearest meaning from the options that are given:

1 'doing drugs' means:
   a. selling drugs.
   b. taking drugs.
   c. making drugs.

2   'acid' is:
a. a chemical compound with hydrogen.
b. LSD.
c. cocaine.

3   'brown' is:
a. amphetamines.
b. crack.
c. heroin.

4   Albert's 'works' are:
a. his job.
b. the factory where he is employed.
c. his equipment.

5   'points' are:
a. needles.
b. money.
c. friends.

6   'the pad' is:
a. his bed.
b. his home.
c. the town he lives in.

7   'it dawned on me' means:
a. in the morning.
b. it happened to me.
c. I realised.

8   'a hit' is:
a. the effect of a drug.
b. a kind of sex.
c. a deep emotional experience.

9   'That was my only time sharing' suggests that Albert Jones contracted HIV from:
a. homosexual sex.
b. sex with the girl he hardly knew.
c. a blood transfusion.
d. a used needle.

Read the medical case study of Albert Jones that follows, which is in a completely different style of language, and answer the questions to help with understanding.

CASE STUDY

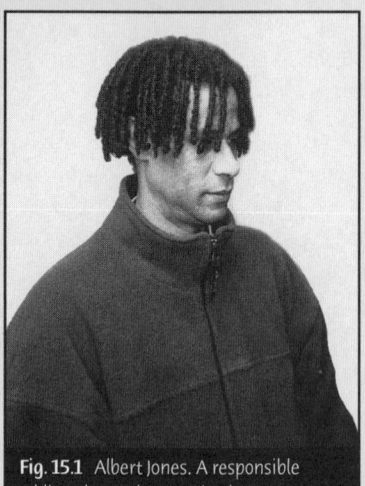

Fig. 15.1 Albert Jones. A responsible addict who made one mistake.

Albert Jones is a 42-year-old male. He has no known drug allergies or intolerances to date.

Medical history

Albert Jones has a history of infections such as:

Pneumocystitis carinii pneumonia (PCP) and oropharyngeal candidiasis.

He has had acquired immune deficiency syndrome (AIDS) since May 1999 and suffers from depression, anaemia and seizures (of unknown origin). The patient also shows symptoms of peripheral neuropathies (i.e. weakness, loss of reflexes and cramps, tingling and numbness in his feet.)

The patient was referred for case conference because he has been receiving suboptimal indinavir doses which have possibly led to an increase in viral load.

Mr Jones began antiretroviral treatment (ARVT) in April 1998 when he was diagnosed with HIV. The doctor was unfamiliar with HIV therapies and prescribed a suboptimal dosage of 200 mg (the recommended dose is 800 mg). Also, the patient took indinavir with food (indinavir should be taken on an empty stomach or with a light meal) and indinavir was administered with phenytoin, a medication for seizures (phenytoin induces an isoenzyme which metabolises indinavir).

The patient was admitted to hospital with PCP. He is very adherent to ARVT.

Though he complains of tingling and numbness in the feet, these do not interfere with activities of daily living.

His depression has improved since treatment with paroxetine.

Recommendations:

1. Consider adding ritonavir 400 mg to current ARVT regime.
2. Add amitriptyline 25 mg for peripheral neuropathy.
3. Draw blood samples at next clinic appointment to measure indinavir and phenytoin concentrations.
4. Patient to attend support-group sessions.

Exercise 15b   **Answer the following questions:**

1 'He has no known drug allergies to date' means that he has no allergies:
   a. up to now.
   b. any longer.
   c. to recently developed medicines.

2 'seizures of unknown origin' are seizures:
   a. we don't know about.
   b. caused by something we don't know about.
   c. which started at a time we are not sure about.

3 'numbness in his feet' is:
a. an inability to walk.
b. a loss of feeling in his feet.
c. pain in his feet.

4 A 'suboptimal' dose is:
a. too much.
b. too little.
c. too late.

5 'The doctor was unfamiliar with HIV therapies' suggests that:
a. the doctor made a mistake.
b. the doctor did not know the patient.
c. the patient made a mistake.

6 When the case study says that 'indinavir was administered with phenytoin', it is suggesting that:
a. phenytoin makes indinavir more effective.
b. indinavir should be taken with phenytoin.
c. phenytoin makes indinavir less effective.

7 'He is very adherent to ARVT' means:
a. the patient likes ARVT.
b. the ARVT is effective.
c. the patient follows the instructions.

8 To '*draw* blood samples' is to:
a. record.
b. take.
c. measure.

Exercise 15c

Choose the correct word from the brackets to complete this summary of Albert Jones' case study:

The patient .... (has, had, has had) AIDS since 1999 and .... (has been, had, used to) suffering from depression, anaemia and seizures. He ...... (was, has, is) been getting an incorrect dosage of indinavir and has been .... (combined, combine, combining) it with food and phenytoin which has .... (made, make, making) it even less effective.

The patient .... (sticking, stuck, sticks) to the recommended treatment at the moment and, despite .... (suffering, suffers, suffered) a variety of illnesses, he ...... (is, can, is able) to continue a relatively normal life. We .... (recommend, recommends, recommending) altering his ARVT regime and carefully .... (monitor, to monitor, monitoring) his progress with regular tests on his blood.

Exercise 15d   Complete the following discharge form for Albert Jones by using the information from above. In each section of the form, choose which option is correct for that section:

DISCHARGE SUMMARY

Date of discharge	Date of admission
10.10.02	23.09.02

Patient	Age
Mr Albert Jones	42 years

PROBLEMS

1 Choose a, b or c:
a. Need for AIDS counselling.
b. Increased dosages of ARVT.
c. Increase of infections (in particular, PCP).

Medical regimen

2 Choose a, b or c:
a. Suboptimal dose of indinavir.
b. Amitriptyline 25 mg + ritonavir 400 mg.
c. Current regimen + drug therapy for peripheral neuropathies.

3 Choose a, b or c:
a. Requires regular monitoring of blood levels.
b. Monitor levels of indinavir & phenytoin.
c. Test for indinavir & phenytoin in blood.

Strengths and resources

4 Choose a, b or c:
a. Adheres to ARVT.
b. Encourage to attend support-group sessions.
c. Tingling and numbness in feet.

Exercise 15e   Rewrite these sentences as if you were giving advice about avoiding HIV infection. The first is done as an example:

a. Don't have unprotected sex with someone who has HIV.
If you have .... you may become infected.

Answer: If you have unprotected sex with someone who has HIV, you may become infected.

b. Don't use a needle or syringe that has already been used by someone else.
If .... you could become infected with HIV.

c. Oral sex with an HIV-infected partner carries a small risk of infection.
If .... there is ....

d. Any contact with blood during sex increases the risk of infection.
If .... the risk of infection ....

e. There is a greater risk of infection with anal intercourse than with vaginal intercourse.

If you have .... of infection is greater than with ....

f. You cannot become infected by kissing someone who has HIV.

If .... infected.

The following sentences are about nursing practices and HIV. Rewrite the sentences beginning with the word(s) given. The first is done as an example:

a. It is assumed that anybody is a potential carrier of a blood-borne virus and so all people in hospital are treated identically.

Assume .... and so treat ....

Answer: Assume that anybody is a potential carrier of a blood-borne virus and so treat all people in hospital identically.

b. Universal precautions are applied whenever there is contact with blood, semen, vaginal secretions or amniotic fluid.

Whenever you have .... apply ....

c. Gloves, protective clothing and eyewear should be used whenever there is a risk of contact with bodily fluids.

Whenever you are at risk ....

d. Spills should be cleaned up with bleach diluted 1:10.

Bleach ....

e. If exposed to HIV, anti-viral treatment should be commenced immediately.

Immediately you .... commence ....

f. HIV can survive within a cadaver (dead body) for up to 16 days.

It is possible ....

g. There is prejudice towards people with HIV even among nurses.

Even some ....

h. A lot of the prejudice is created by wrong information.

Wrong ....

i. A nurse cannot refuse to care for a person with HIV or AIDS.

It is not possible ....

Chemical happiness

This is an account by a young man of the time he overdosed on the drug Ecstasy.

I reckon Ecstasy is a wonderful drug. It brings feelings of overwhelming happiness and love but I've got to say that too much chemical happiness can affect your ability to be happy for real.

For three years now I've been taking Ecstasy. I used to drop a couple of Es every Friday and then three or four on Saturdays. I needed more on Saturday to bring me back to the same level as Friday.

After a year of this, things began to deteriorate and I realised I was becoming dependant. I would be depressed during the week and feel very wound up with sleepless nights and anxiety attacks. I was put on Prozac, started to get pains around the kidneys and my memory was all in pieces. I tried to cut down my use of Es and stopped hanging out with mates that take them.

But recently I went to a rave and when I was there decided to double drop. Don't ask me why, I know it was a mistake. Anyway, within 25 minutes I began to feel euphoric but it came on too strong. I was sick all over my tee-shirt and I got this picture-frame vision where everything gets frozen.

I got worried and so I went over to the first-aid tent. There were two male nurses there and I told them I had overdosed. One of them sneered and said I was 'an idiot in dreamland'. This just made me annoyed.

They sat me down and made me take off my tee-shirt and gave me a glass of water to drink. The nice one told me to sip it or I would be sick again. I went into a kind of trance and for the next couple of days I was a wreck – paranoid as hell, shaking and with involuntary muscle spasms.

I reckon now that if I hadn't been sick then something worse would have happened to me. I am careful now. I mean, you've got to be careful or you just end up freaking out.

Exercise 15g

Replace the colloquialisms in brackets in the following sentences with a more standard English expression from a, b or c.

1 'I used to (drop) a couple of Es every Friday.'
a. buy
b. inject
c. swallow

2 'I stopped (hanging out) with mates who take Es.'
a. going around with
b. shopping
c. playing

3 'I decided to (double drop).'
  a. overdose.
  b. halve my usual amount.
  c. take twice as much as usual.

4 You end up (freaking out).
  a. going mad.
  b. dying.
  c. running around.

Exercise 15h

This is a formal report based upon what the young man has said. Fill in the spaces by selecting the correct word from each of the brackets.

The patient has been a regular drug .... (abuse, abusive, abuser) and reports he has been taking MDMA (Ecstasy) for the past three years. During this period he has noticed that his general mental health has become .... (impaired, impair, impairment). This impairment includes a general .... (confusion, confused, confuse), insomnia, depersonalisation and paranoid .... (psychosis, psychotic, psychology).

Studies have indeed shown that MDMA use is related to a (lower, lowering, low) of serotonin, which is associated with depression and .... (anxiety, anxious, anxiously). Severe chronic anxiety can be treated with diazepam, fluoxetine or sertraline, insomnia with temazepam and panic attacks with lorazepam. However, because all of these drugs are potentially .... (addictive, addiction, addict), the patient's GP thought it best to use an antidepressant for no more than .... (a few, few, fewer) weeks.

Unfortunately, the patient returned to using the drug whilst at a 'rave' where he took twice his normal intake of MDMA and was .... (overwhelming, overwhelm, overwhelmed) by the combined effect of the drug and the mesmeric, trance- .... (induce, induction, inducing) music and psychedelic visuals. He experienced .... (hallucinate, hallucinations, hallucinated) and vomited. The patient then reported to the first-aid facility for assistance, where unfortunately he experienced a judgmental attitude from staff. This was particularly unhelpful because this young man has .... (difficult, difficulties, a difficult) with authority figures and he became unco-operative and eventually refused the assistance that was offered.

The patient does not show the typical .... (denial, deny, denying) defence mechanisms of many MDMA users and there is reason to believe that he will be able to successfully .... (withdraw, withdrawal, withdrew) from the drug without the help of antipsychotics such as haloperidol.

Exercise 15i

The UK public's attitude to HIV/AIDS

These are the results of a survey of people in the UK about their attitudes and beliefs about AIDS. (MORI poll 1.12.2000) Each line of the list has a letter (A–G). After the list there is a chart which gives the same information but the chart is not labelled. Label each part of the chart with the appropriate letter (A–G).

A. 1 in 10 people wrongly believe that there is a cure for AIDS.

B. 14% of the population are happy to give money to AIDS research.

C. Nine out of ten adults know that sex is the main cause of HIV infection.

D. 57% of the population believe that people who become infected only have themselves to blame.

E. 75% of the population get their information about HIV from television soap operas like 'Eastenders' rather than official sources like government information leaflets.

F. 1 in 4 adults believe they don't know enough about the risks of HIV.

G. Two-thirds of the UK population have made no change to their lifestyle in response to the dangers of HIV/AIDS.

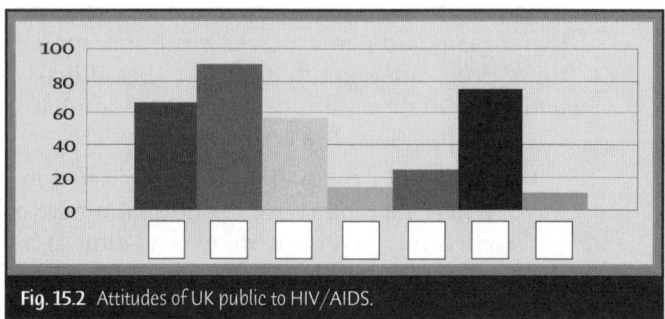

Fig. 15.2 Attitudes of UK public to HIV/AIDS.

Exercise 15i: Further practice

Read the notes about a patient who, like Mr Jones, receives nursing care at home and complete the form that follows:

Henry Macdonald is 63. One afternoon he suddenly became aware of weakness in his right side. He began to dribble saliva, his vision became blurred and he found he was not able to call out for help. The doctor diagnosed a cerebrovascular accident with right-sided hemiplegia.

Mr Macdonald is overweight – he weighs 15 stones (95 kg). A desirable weight for a man of his build is between 72 and 81 kg. In discussion with the patient, it is decided that his aim must be to lose 6 kg every month. This means the District Nurse must supervise a daily diet of 4200 kilojoules (1000 calories). Also, Mr Macdonald needs help with his expressive aphasia. For example, he should be shown lip and tongue exercises and be given encouragement to read aloud.

Patient:		
Medical diagnosis:		
Patient's problems	Goals	Nursing instructions

Answers and comments on the language

Exercise 15a

1 b.

2 b.

3 c. There is a big vocabulary connected to illegal drugs and a lot of the words are international. These are just a few of them: cocaine is called 'snow', 'bump', 'candy' or 'toot'. Ecstasy is called 'E'. When cocaine is sniffed it is 'snorted' and when heroin smoke is sniffed it is called 'chasing the dragon'. The vocabulary comes in and out of fashion and new words are being added all the time.

4 c.

5 a.

6 b. The town you live in is sometimes called 'your patch'.

7 c.

8 a.

9 d.

Exercise 15b

1 a. 'Date' can be a verb. 'To date' something is to say how old it is (an antique, for example) but 'to date' someone is to go out with them. If something is 'dated' it is old fashioned, whereas if something is 'up to date' it is modern and recent. If someone is 'up to date' they have the most recent information.

2 b. Note the use of the word 'of' here as in: 'a cyst of unknown size' or: 'an attack of unknown duration' (i.e. we don't know how long the attack went on for).

3 b. See previous chapters for uses of the word 'numb'.

4 b. The prefix 'sub' means 'under' so 'suboptimal' means 'under the most effective level'.

5   a.

6   c.

7   c. 'Adhere' means 'stick to' (as in 'adhesive').

8   b.

Exercise 15c

The patient <u>has had</u> AIDS since 1999 and <u>has been</u> suffering from depression, anaemia and seizures. He <u>has</u> been getting an incorrect dosage of indinavir and has been <u>combining</u> it with food and phenytoin which has <u>made</u> it even less effective.

The patient <u>sticks</u> to the recommended treatment at the moment and despite <u>suffering</u> a variety of illnesses, he <u>is able</u> to continue a relatively normal life. We <u>recommend</u> altering his ARVT regime and carefully monitoring his progress with regular tests on his blood.

Exercise 15d

DISCHARGE SUMMARY	
Date of discharge 10.10.02	**Date of admission** 23.09.02
Patient Mr Albert Jones	**Age** 42 years

PROBLEMS

1 The correct answer is **c.** Option **a** is not a 'problem' but a 'requirement' or a 'need'. Option **b** is a 'recommendation'.

Medical regimen

2 The correct answer is **b.** Option **a** is incomplete and does not totally describe the new regimen. Option **a** is in fact a 'problem' which describes the patient's previous medical regimen.

3 The correct answer is **b.** Option **a** suggests monitoring quantities of blood rather than what is in the blood. Option **c** suggests testing the blood to find out if indinavir and phenytoin are in the blood – which we know already.

Strengths and resources

4 The best answer is **a.** Option **b** is a 'recommendation'. Option **c** is a 'problem'.

Exercise 15e

b. If you use a needle or syringe that has already been used by someone else, you could become infected with HIV.

c. If you have oral sex with an HIV infected partner, there is a small risk of infection.

d. If you have contact with blood during sex, the risk of infection increases.

e. If you have anal intercourse, the risk of infection is greater than with vaginal intercourse.

f. If you kiss someone who has HIV, you cannot become infected.

Exercise 15f

b. Whenever you have contact with blood, semen, vaginal fluids or amniotic fluid, apply universal precautions.

c. Whenever you are at risk of contact with bodily fluids, use gloves, protective clothing and eyewear.

d. Bleach diluted 1:10 should be used to clean up spills.

e. Immediately you are exposed to HIV, (you should) commence antiviral treatment.

f. It is possible for HIV to survive within a cadaver for up to 16 days.

g. Even some nurses are prejudiced towards people with HIV.

h. Wrong information creates a lot of the prejudice.

i. It is not possible for a nurse to refuse to care for a person with HIV or AIDS.

Exercise 15g

1 c.

2 a. Variations on this expression include 'hanging about', 'chilling out', 'hanging around', etc.

3 c.

4 a. 'To freak out' can also mean 'to get angry'. A freak is a strange person or 'not normal'. A 'freak storm', for example, refers to unusual weather, a 'freak accident' is an unusual and completely unexpected accident.

Exercise 15h

The patient has been a regular drug <u>abuser</u> and reports he has been taking MDMA (Ecstasy) for the past three years. During this period, he has noticed that his general mental health has become <u>impaired</u>. This impairment includes a general <u>confusion</u>, insomnia, depersonalisation and paranoid <u>psychosis</u>.

Studies have indeed shown that MDMA use is related to a <u>lowering</u> of serotonin, which is associated with depression and <u>anxiety</u>. Severe chronic anxiety can be treated with diazepam, fluoxetine or sertraline, insomnia with temazepam and panic attacks with lorazepam. However, because all of these drugs are potentially <u>addictive</u>, the patient's GP thought it best to use an antidepressant for no more than <u>a few</u> weeks.

Unfortunately the patient returned to using the drug whilst at a 'rave' where he took twice his normal intake of MDMA and was <u>overwhelmed</u> by the combined effect of the drug and the mesmeric, trance-<u>inducing</u> music and psychedelic visuals. He experienced <u>hallucinations</u> and vomited. The patient then reported to the first-aid facility for assistance where unfortunately he experienced a judgmental attitude from staff. This was particularly unhelpful because this young man has <u>difficulties</u> with authority figures and he became unco-operative and eventually refused the assistance that was offered.

The patient does not show the typical <u>denial</u> defence mechanisms of many MDMA users and there is reason to believe that he will be able to successfully <u>withdraw</u> from the drug without the help of antipsychotics such as haloperidol.

Exercise 15i

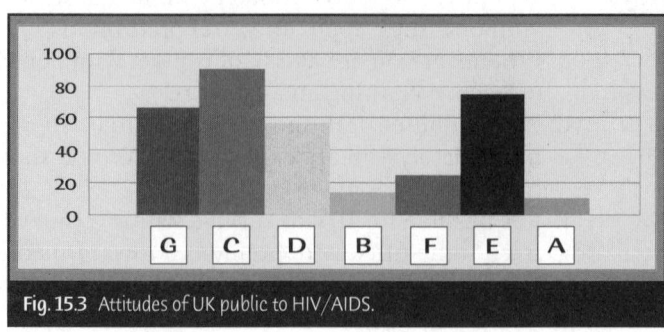

Fig. 15.3 Attitudes of UK public to HIV/AIDS.

Exercise 15i: Further practice

Patient
Mr Henry Macdonald

Medical diagnosis:
Cerebrovascular accident with right sided hemiplegia.

Patient's problems	Goals	Nursing intervention
Overweight	Reduce weight from 95 kg to 72–81 kg (reduced by 6 kg monthly)	Supervise 4200 kJ diet
Expressive aphasia	Speaking intelligibly	Teach lip and tongue exercises Encourage to read aloud.

Part Three

Talking and listening

Chapter Sixteen

About communicating with patients

Listening to patients

Because an important part of a nurse's work is communicating with patients, nurses don't just need to understand medical terminology, they also need to understand the dialects, accents and idioms that patients use.

Speech is very different from writing and across countries like the UK the speech of people can vary enormously and present anybody, even native speakers, with problems of understanding.

Here is a conversation between two women in a GP's waiting room in Bristol (south-west England). The conversation is written as it sounds so it illustrates the sort of difficulties you face when you know the language but you don't know the accent. (Adapted from *Son of Bristol* by Vic Wiltshire)

FIRST WOMAN: Ear, oi thaw chewed sed chewunt come near namore. Chew sed thes doc trad coal dans, din chew?

SECOND WOMAN: Ar, buthawaur lass cheer. It be diffrun now, they gotta new doctrine ear annes a goodun ee is. Is answer warms toast.

TRANSLATION:

FIRST WOMAN: Here, I thought you said you weren't coming here anymore. You said this doctor had cold hands, didn't you?

SECOND WOMAN: Yes, but that was last year. It's different now, they've got a new doctor in here and he's a good one, he is. His hands are as warm as toast.

Understanding what patients say is not always as difficult as this example. Here is something comparatively easy.

This is a conversation between a nurse and a Mrs Jakes, who is being admitted to hospital. The nurse needs some basic information from the patient in order to complete an admission form and a care plan. The patient uses a lot of idioms.

NURSE: I've just got one or two questions to ask you, Mrs Jakes – it won't take long. OK?

MRS JAKES: OK nurse.

NURSE: The first one is er … yes, just here, right. Do you see a District Nurse or Social Worker at home?

MRS JAKES: Sometimes a nurse drops in.

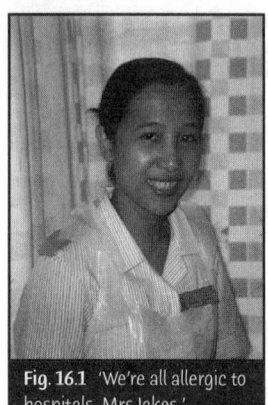

NURSE: And how often do you see her?

MRS JAKES: About <u>once every couple a weeks or so</u>.

NURSE: Do you get Meals on Wheels or Home Help?

MRS JAKES: No dear. I don't need no help thank you.

NURSE: Who's your GP, Mrs Jakes?

MRS JAKES: Dr McDonald.

NURSE: Are you allergic to anything?

MRS JAKES: Nothing as far as I know. Oh, hospitals – I'm allergic to hospitals! [laughs]

NURSE: [laughs] Aren't we all? <u>How long have you been feeling poorly?</u>

MRS JAKES: <u>Been coming on about three months now</u>, four more likely. I went to see Dr McDonald three months ago, in June, it was.

NURSE: Do you have any problems with your health other than these pains in your chest?

MRS JAKES: Got varicose veins – don't half hurt when I walk around.

NURSE: What did Dr McDonald tell you was the reason for you coming into hospital?

MRS JAKES: 'Investigation', he said. They want to find out what's causing the pain in me chest.

NURSE: Has the doctor given you any idea of how long you will be in hospital?

MRS JAKES: Couldn't tell, he said. Could be a short stay, he said.

NURSE: Do you have a job?

MRS JAKES: I'm a cleaner, dear, just part-time, you know, couple of evenings a week at the primary school in Green Street.

NURSE: Have you got any children?

MRS JAKES: There's George, he's in the army away in Cyprus at the moment and Sarah – she's a nurse, just like you, dear.

NURSE: Do you have anyone else you have to look after at home?

MRS JAKES: No dear, there's just meself and Henry the canary.

NURSE: <u>Is there a Mr Jakes?</u>

MRS JAKES: No. He died couple a year back.

NURSE: Are there any problems at home because you are in hospital?

MRS JAKES: There's Henry. I've got her at number 33 to come in. She'll feed the bird and get my pension. People are nice sometimes, aren't they?

NURSE: Yes. Are you on any special diet, Mrs Jakes?

MRS JAKES: No, nothing special, but the doctor says I've got to cut down cholesterol.

NURSE: OK, so no chips? Is there any food you don't like?

MRS JAKES: No, eat anything me – except beetroot. I hate beetroot. Always reminds me...

NURSE: ...of school dinners [laughs]. Yes, me too. Do you have a good appetite?

MRS JAKES: Normally eat like a horse, but been going off me food recently.

NURSE: What about sleeping, how many hours do you usually sleep at night?

MRS JAKES: Any little thing wakes me up these days. Used to sleep like a log, not any more though. It's the pain you see – keeps me awake and then if I get to doze off it wakes me up this pain here and here. <u>I'd love a good night's sleep</u>. Forgotten what it's like.

NURSE: Do you normally have to take any tablets to make you sleep?

MRS JAKES: Dr McDonald gave me them [shakes box of tablets] – not much good though.

NURSE: Bowels OK? Any problems? How often do you open your bowels?

MRS JAKES: Me what, love?

NURSE: <u>Big toilet</u>. You know. Have you done it today? Have you opened your bowels today?

MRS JAKES: Used to be regular as clockwork. But lately been having trouble with constipation – really painful sometimes.

NURSE: Do you take anything for it? – the constipation?

MRS JAKES: Ex-Lax seems to work all right.

NURSE: Do you have any problems passing water? Do you have to get up in the night to pass water?

MRS JAKES: No, I used to be all right there but recently, as I say, I've been having problems and sometimes I'm up and down all night long. It does make me fed up.

NURSE: Do you have periods any more?

MRS JAKES: No dear – stopped about seven or eight year ago.

NURSE: How's your hearing? No problem there, I think?

MRS JAKES: No fine, hearing's right as rain. Eyes getting worse though, need a new pair of <u>specs</u> I suppose.

NURSE: Do you wear dentures?

MRS JAKES: Yes.

NURSE: Are they top or bottom?

MRS JAKES: Both, dear, both top and bottom I'm afraid. <u>It's rotten getting old</u> isn't it?

Exercise 16a

Say which of the following statements are true:

a. When Mrs Jakes says she gets a visit from a nurse 'once every couple a weeks or so', she means the nurse comes at the same time every two weeks.

b. When the nurse asks Mrs Jakes how long she has been 'poorly', she wants to know about Mrs Jakes' income.

c. When the patient says 'it's been coming on about three months now', she means the pain has gradually increased.

d. When the nurse says 'Is there a Mr Jakes?', she is asking if Mrs Jakes has a son.

e. Mrs Jakes says 'I'd love a good night's sleep'. This means she enjoys going to bed.

f. When the nurse mentions 'big toilet', she is asking about the equipment in Mrs Jakes' bathroom.

g. Mrs Jakes needs a new pair of 'specs' because she is going deaf.

h. When Mrs Jakes says 'it's rotten getting old', she is referring to the way that teeth decay as you get older.

Exercise 16b   Most of what Mrs Jakes says is fairly easy to understand, though
you may not know some of the expressions she uses. However,
the idioms are logical and you can probably work out what they
mean. Here are some of the things she says. Choose an expression
from a, b and c that means the same thing as the idiom.

1   A nurse 'drops in':
a. lets something slip out of her hand.
b. calls at the patient's house.
c. makes an appointment before calling.

2   'I don't need no help'.
a. I need help.
b. I get no help.
c. I don't need any help.

3   Varicose veins 'don't half hurt'.
a. hurt a lot.
b. don't hurt much.
c. hurt only half as much as they used to.

4   'I eat like a horse'.
a. I like horsemeat.
b. I am a vegetarian.
c. I eat a lot.

5   'I'm going off' my food.
a. I've got no appetite.
b. My food is bad.
c. I don't like my food.

6   I used to 'sleep like a log'.
a. sleep badly.
b. sleep often.
c. sleep deeply.

7   I used to be 'regular as clockwork'.
a. always at the same time.
b. never late.
c. always early.

8   Any problems 'passing water'?
a. drinking
b. swimming
c. urinating

9   I'm 'up and down'.
a. restless.
b. get out of bed a lot.
c. happy and then unhappy.

10   My hearing is 'right as rain'.
a. poor.
b. no problem.
c. OK in bad weather.

Exercise 16c   Using the information from the conversation with Mrs Jakes, fill in the following admission form:

PATIENT ADMISSION FORM

PERSONAL DETAILS

Name: Mrs Susan Jakes   **Next of kin:**

Address: 33, Duck Lane,
              Moreton,
              Devon

Name of GP:

Patient's understanding of admission:

MEDICAL INFORMATION

Relevant medical history:

Allergies:

Bowels:

Urinary:

(Female patients) Menstruation:

Hearing:

Vision:

Oral:

Talking to patients

It is now common practice for nurses to communicate with patients as much as possible when they are doing routine nursing tasks. If nurses talk, the patients become involved in their treatment.

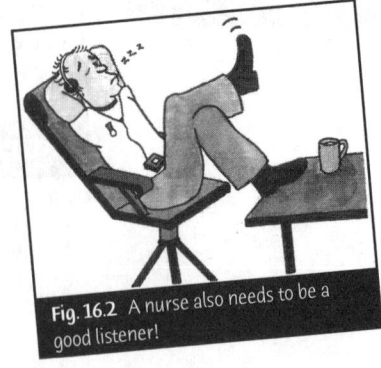

Fig. 16.2 A nurse also needs to be a good listener!

Here is an example of a nurse talking to a patient as she takes the patient's blood pressure. You will see how the nurse says what she is going to do, explains why she is doing it and gives the patient feedback.

NURSE: Mrs Jackson, I'm just going to do some routine tests. I want to start off with your blood pressure. Just to make sure that everything's OK. All right?

MRS JACKSON: I see, yes of course.

NURSE: So, I'm going to wrap this around your arm then I'll pump some air into it so I can read your blood pressure ...... how's that feel? OK?

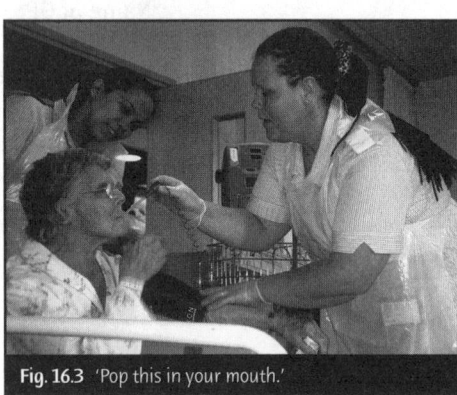

Fig. 16.3 'Pop this in your mouth.'

MRS JACKSON: Feels a bit funny.

NURSE: Does it? Never mind, it'll be over in a second or two.

MRS JACKSON: Is it OK? My pressure I mean?

NURSE: Yes, everything's perfectly normal. Right as rain. Now we'll just take your temperature. Can you pop this in your mouth, under your tongue? Good. And while you're doing that I'll just take your pulse.

Below are step-by-step training instructions to nurses for how to give a bedbath. Under each line of the instructions is an example of what the nurse would say to the patient.

a. Patients may need a bedbath if they are extremely weak.
NURSE: You're probably not strong enough to bathe yourself at the moment, so I'm going to give you a bedbath.

b. Ensure the patient's privacy by drawing the curtains round their bed.
NURSE: I'll draw the curtains so that we can be private.

c. Use a sheet to cover the parts of the patient not being washed.
NURSE: I'll use this sheet to cover you up as I go.

d. Start with patient's face, ears and neck.
NURSE: I'll start with your face and work downwards.

e. Ask the patient if they would like to use their own toiletries and talcum powder.
NURSE: Shall I use your own talcum powder? Is that OK?

Exercise 16d

Now do the same thing with these instructions for syringing an ear – at each stage write down what you would say to the patient.

a. Before you start, ask the patient to tell you if at any time they feel any pain.

....

b. Examine inside the patient's ear (external canal and eardrum) with an auriscope.

....

c. Fill the syringe with the warm fluid.

....

d. Place a protective covering over the patient's shoulder.

....

e. Pull the pinna of the ear upwards and back to straighten out the canal.

....

f. Send a jet of the fluid into the ear to clear it out.

....

Exercise 16e

The following article is about the therapeutic value of talking with patients. Fill in the spaces in the text with the correct word(s) from the brackets.

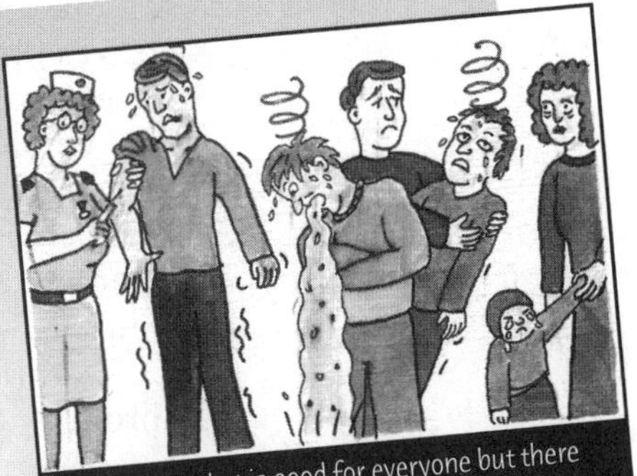

Fig. 16.4 A chat is good for everyone but there may not always be time for a long conversation.

TALKING IS GOOD FOR YOU

Medical research in America and the UK shows that communicating is an important part of medical .... (treatment, treated, treating) and that opportunities for patients to talk .... (on, with, about) their illnesses have a significant .... (effectiveness, effective, effect) on the success of treatment and the .... (speed, velocity, rapid) of recovery.

In America, research into .... (man, male, masculine) patients recovering from heart bypass surgery showed that patients who could .... (share, shared, sharing) their thoughts and fears with other men in a similar situation were less .... (anxiety, anxiously, anxious), more active and were .... (discharged, discharge, discharging) from hospital sooner than those treated in .... (isolated, isolation, isolate).

Also in the US, research into women .... (had, with, who) breast cancer shows that patients .... (do, have, go) better after treatment if they .... (make, get, do) a chance to talk about their fears. Talking and listening to patients has the effect .... (to, of, with) reducing the amount of medical appointments .... (of, for, with) problems associated with their cancer. A spokesman for the organisation Cancer Bacup said in an interview with the BBC, 'discussing the situation can benefit a .... (patient, patients, patient's) sense of well-being.'

Research in Scotland into the effect of providing breast cancer patients with the support of specialist nurses who encourage their patients to talk about their illness showed similar results. Talking helped patients .... (coping, cope, coped) psychologically and .... (positive, positively, a positive) affected their rate of recovery.

Exercise 16f

As a contrast of styles read this conversation in which a nurse is talking to a patient who is worried about incontinence. Complete the text by choosing the correct word from each of the brackets.

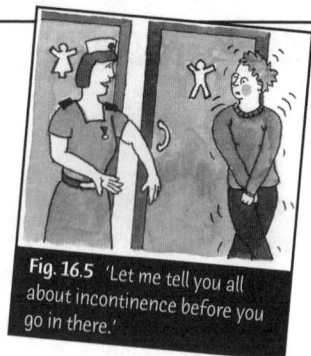

Fig. 16.5 'Let me tell you all about incontinence before you go in there.'

'One .... (causing, cause, cased) of your leaking might be what's sitting in your medicine cupboard right now. It could be your medicines. Do you know how it all works? Your bladder, I mean? Well it goes like this: your bladder .... (storage, stores, store) your urine, right? It's like a .... (ballooning, balloon, balloonist) and as it fills up the muscles .... (relax, relaxing, relaxed) and then when you want to spend a penny, the muscles tighten up and .... (squeezing, squeezes, squeeze) the urine out.

You've got your urethra, which is a tube, and the urine leaves the bladder through this tube – this urethra. With me so far? There's another muscle that .... (keep, keeps, keeping) the urethra closed. It's a bit like a rubber band. Then when you go to the toilet, your brain .... (speaks to, says, tells) the bladder to tighten up and then the urine leaves through the urethra. So you've got all these things .... (work, works, working) together – bladder, urethra, muscles and nerves and the whole system's got to work. But it doesn't always work efficiently. You can get .... (leak, leaked, leaking), you see, caused by your medicines. You have high blood pressure, don't you? Yes, well, medicines to treat high blood pressure sometimes make the sphincter muscles – the ones around the urethra – sometimes they make them too .... (loosen, loosely, loose) and then the urethra doesn't close properly and you get .... (leak, some leak, a leak).

There is an obvious remedy – you stop taking the medicines – but in your case I think there may be no alternative – you've got to keep ...... (take, to take, taking) them. There are exercises you can do ...... (training, train, to train) your muscles to work better. I can show you these if you like. But don't stop taking the medicine until .... (you've, you, you'll) talked to the doctor.

There are other things. Do you drink a lot of coffee? Coffee can .... (take, give, have) you problems – or chocolate even. Alcohol of course. So you see there are all sorts of causes and no you're not .... (having, going, coming) senile and I know it's .... (embarrassment, embarrassed, embarrassing) but this sort of thing affects all sorts of people. You'd be .... (amazing, amaze, amazed) by how many people suffer from it.

And I know there's a stigma .... (attach, attaching, attached) to incontinence though there's absolutely nothing to be .... (ashamed, a shame, shameful) of. Tell you what, when's your next appointment with your GP? Well, put together a list of all the medicines you .... (taking, took, take) and when you see the doctor ask him if any of them can cause bladder problems and then .... (say, talk, tell) him what you've .... (said, spoke, told) me.'

Euphemisms

A euphemism is a substitute for another word which might be offensive or hurtful. Because medical staff have to deal with things which are often embarrassing or difficult to talk about – toileting, sex, death and so on – they often use euphemisms to be properly understood by patients or to ease both patient and nurse through difficult or potentially awkward moments.

The euphemism you use often depends on the person you are talking to. Instead of the word 'penis' you might use the word 'willy' (see below) when talking to a boy, but probably not when talking to a middle-aged man. Here are some examples you commonly hear in UK hospitals:

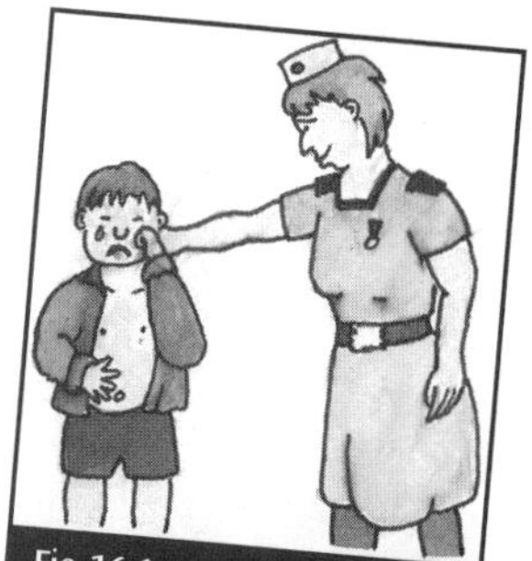

Fig. 16.6 'You say your tummy hurts around your belly button?'

VOCABULARY

stomach: tummy, tum, belly. The navel is often referred to as a 'belly button'. The fat around the stomach is sometimes called 'the spare tyre'.

to urinate: many euphemisms including to spend a penny, to pass water, to have a pee, to piss, to wee, to have a wee, to have a Jimmy Riddle, to piddle, number ones. 'To piss' is fairly vulgar. The urinary system is sometimes called 'the waterworks'.

to defecate: to move/open bowels, to pass a motion, to shit, (do) big ones, number two(s), to poo, to do a poo.' 'To shit' is vulgar.

buttocks/anus: bottom, bum, arse, botty, butt, back-end, derriere, back bottom. 'Arse' and 'butt' are vulgar and best avoided.

genitals: two general euphemisms for genitals applied to both men and women are 'bits' and 'private parts' as in: 'here's a flannel to wipe your bits/private parts'. A penis is referred to by different people in different situations as: prick, dick, willy, John Thomas, member, organ, etc. An aroused penis is usually called an 'erection'. Testicles are often referred to as 'balls' and sometimes 'cods', 'nuts,' etc. All of these words should be used with care and are best avoided. Use the word 'testicles'.

to die: to pass away, to pass on, to go to (your) maker, to be deceased. Expressions that make light of death include: 'to kick the bucket', 'to push up daisies', 'to pop (your) clogs', 'to snuff it', etc.

Exercise 16g

The following sentences contain euphemisms and idioms. Choose from a, b and c which is closest in meaning to each sentence:

1 'How are the waterworks, Mrs Brown?'
a. 'Is it raining outside?'
b. 'Do you have any problems with urinating?'
c. 'Do you know anything about plumbing?'

2 'Is it painful when you pass water?'
a. 'Does it hurt when you urinate?'
b. 'Does it hurt to wash?'
c. 'Are you afraid of drowning?'

3 'It hurts every time I open my bowels.'
a. 'A rectum examination is painful.'
b. 'I have constipation.'
c. 'It's painful when I go to the toilet.'

4 'Wee in this bottle.'
a. 'Drink a little of this.'
b. 'There's a little bit in this bottle.'
c. 'Use this bottle for your urine.'

5 'Have you got rid of that spare tyre?'
a. 'Have you lost weight?'
b. 'Have you repaired your car?'
c. 'You look fatter.'

Communication errors

Exercise 16h

Here are some real-life examples of mistakes in vocabulary or grammar which have occurred in hospitals. They are meant to be humorous but if you don't see the joke it is probably because you don't immediately see the grammatical mistake or misunderstanding which makes them funny. Read them and see if you can identify what exactly is going wrong. Explanations are in the Answers section.

a. 'What brought you to the clinic?' asked a nurse wanting to put the patient at ease. The patient answered: 'We borrowed a car.'

b. A doctor walked into the records department looking for a Mr Wilson's medical records. He couldn't find them at first and left. Suddenly the clerk discovered the file and ran after the doctor calling 'Mr Wilson's history!' Mr Wilson was being wheeled down the hall on a trolley. He sat upright and cried, 'I didn't know a broken ankle was that serious!'

c. 'In a couple of days, the knee will be better and after three days it will completely disappear.'

d. 'The patient has been depressed ever since she began seeing me in 1983.'

e. 'The patient's discharge status is: alive but without permission.'

f. 'The patient refused an autopsy.'

g. 'The patient doesn't have a past history of suicides.'

h. 'The patient has chest pain if she lies on her left side for over a year.'

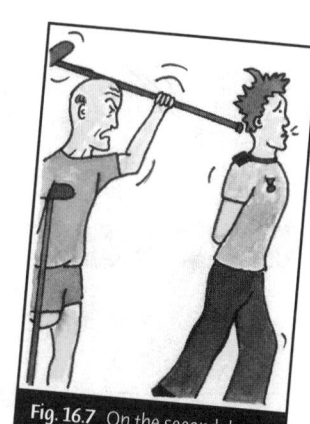

Fig. 16.7 On the second day, the knee was better and on the third day it had completely disappeared.

Answers and comments on the language

Exercise 16a

a. is not true. If she had said 'once every couple a weeks' then maybe she would have meant that the visits are fairly regular. Even so, the word 'couple' instead of 'two' suggests a vagueness about the timing. The important details here are the words 'or so', which mean 'roughly', 'approximately' or 'about'. 'Fifty metres or so' means 'about fifty metres' or 'perhaps a bit more than fifty metres'.

b. is not true. 'Feeling poorly' means 'feeling ill'. However 'to be poor' is to have little money, 'to be poorly dressed' is to be dressed badly – in old, dirty clothes. 'Driving poorly' means 'driving badly'.

c. is true. 'Coming on' here means 'gradually increasing/building up'. 'It's been coming on to rain for the past two days' means the clouds have been building up for the past two days.

d. is not true. 'A Mr Jakes' is her husband. Also, if you want Mr William Brown and you don't know which one he is in a crowded waiting room, you might call, 'Is there <u>a</u> Mr William Brown here?'

e. is not true. She means that she can't sleep properly and deeply at night. You do not hear people say 'A good day's sleep.' However, people do say 'a good day's work', meaning 'a job well done'.

f. is not true. In this chapter there is a section on medical euphemisms and one euphemism for defecating is 'big toilet'. You 'go to' or 'do' big toilet.

g. is not true. 'Specs' is short for spectacles, glasses.

h. is not true. 'Rotten' expresses something unpleasant or bad. 'He's a rotten doctor' means 'he is a bad doctor'. 'This is a rotten experience' means 'this is a bad experience.' In the expression 'it's rotten getting old', 'it' doesn't refer to anything any more than it does in 'it's raining'.

Exercise 16b

1 b. 'To drop in' is to call on someone usually without a prior arrangement or appointment. A 'drop-in clinic' is a clinic where you don't normally need an appointment.

2 c. Logically, she should mean 'I need help' because of the two negatives in this sentence and in mathematics two negatives make a positive. But two negatives are common in colloquial UK English and they don't create a positive meaning. For example 'I don't want no potatoes' means 'I don't want potatoes'. 'I haven't got no money' means 'I have got no money'.

3 a. 'don't/won't/haven't' + 'half' expresses emphasis. 'I wouldn't half like a beer' means 'I would love a beer'. 'I don't half like you' means 'I like you a lot.'

4 c. Similar to this expression is 'I could eat a horse' which means 'I am hungry'. Horse words and expressions are still in common use in English obviously dating from before the motor car. Others include: 'to work like a horse' (to work hard), 'don't look a gift horse in the mouth' (don't criticise presents), 'to horse about' (to mess around), 'to have horse sense' (to be sensible).

5   a. To 'go off' someone or something is to no longer like them/it. Things like food can 'go off' meaning they start to decay and go bad. 'This milk has gone off' means 'the milk has gone bad'.

6   c. There are a number of expressions which mean to sleep deeply. 'To sleep like a log', 'to sleep like a dog', 'to sleep like a baby', 'to sleep like the dead' are some of them.

7   a. 'To be regular' often refers to bowel movements and periods.

8   c. 'To pass water' is a euphemism for 'urinating' (see Euphemisms).

9   b. The answer could be option **a** (restless). But in this case Mrs Jakes is referring to waking up and going to the toilet.

10   b. There are a lot of expressions which mean 'good', 'perfect', for example; 'hunkey dorey', 'spot on', 'bostin' (Midlands English), 'A1', 'ace', 'beaut', 'dead smart', 'top drawer', etc.

Exercise 16c

PATIENT ADMISSION FORM

PERSONAL DETAILS

Name: Mrs Susan Jakes   **Next of kin:** George Jakes (son)
Address: 33, Duck Lane,
           Moreton,
           Devon

Name of GP:
Dr McDonald

Patient's understanding of admission:
Investigation of chest pains

MEDICAL INFORMATION

Relevant medical history:
Varicose veins
Pains in chest increasing over past three months

Allergies:
None

Bowels:
Suffers from constipation, takes Ex-Lax

Urinary:
Urinates a lot, especially at night – interferes with sleep

(Female patients) Menstruation:
Periods stopped 7/8 years ago

Hearing:
OK

Vision:
Wears glasses

Oral:
Wears dentures – upper and lower.

Exercise 16d

There will of course be many variations to the answers in this exercise so the following are a few examples of good ones.

a. Let me know at any time if there is any pain.
or: Tell me if you feel any pain at any time.
or: This shouldn't hurt, but if it does let me know straight away.

b. I'm going to use this and have a look inside your ear.
or: I'll just have a look inside your ear with this.
or: This is an auriscope and I'm going to use it to look inside your ear.

c. I'm going to fill the syringe with warm fluid.
or: I'm going to squirt warm fluid into your ear to wash it out.

d. I'll just put this over your shoulder to save you from getting wet.
or: I'm putting a cover over your shoulder so you don't get wet.

e. I'm going to pull your ear back a bit so that the water goes directly in.
or: I'm just pulling your ear back a little to straighten out the inside of your ear so that the water goes all the way in.

f. You're going to feel the water rush into your ear. It shouldn't be too unpleasant.
or: You're going to feel the water going into your ear.
or: I'm going to squirt the water into your ear now.

Exercise 16e

Medical research in America and the UK shows that communicating is an important part of medical <u>treatment</u> and that opportunities for patients to talk <u>about</u> their illnesses have a significant <u>effect</u> on the success of treatment and the <u>speed</u> of recovery.

In America, research into <u>male</u> patients recovering from heart bypass surgery showed that patients who could <u>share</u> their thoughts and fears with other men in a similar situation were less <u>anxious</u>, more active and were <u>discharged</u> from hospital sooner than those treated in <u>isolation</u>.

Also in the US, research into women <u>with</u> breast cancer shows that patients <u>do</u> better after treatment if they <u>get</u> a chance to talk about their fears. Talking and listening to patients has the effect <u>of</u> reducing the amount of medical appointments <u>for</u> problems associated with their cancer. A spokesman for the organisation Cancer Bacup said in an interview with the BBC, 'discussing the situation can benefit a <u>patient's</u> sense of well-being.'

Research in Scotland into the effect of providing breast cancer patients with the support of specialist nurses who encourage their patients to talk about their illness showed similar results. Talking helped patients <u>cope</u> psychologically and <u>positively</u> affected their rate of recovery.

Exercise 16f

'One <u>cause</u> of your leaking might be what's sitting in your medicine cupboard right now. It could be your medicines. Do you know how it all works? Your bladder, I mean? Well it goes like this: your bladder <u>stores</u> your urine, right? It's like a <u>balloon</u> and as it fills up the muscles <u>relax</u> and then when you want to spend a penny, the muscles tighten up and <u>squeeze</u> the urine out.

You've got your urethra, which is a tube, and the urine leaves the bladder through this tube – this urethra. With me so far? There's another muscle that <u>keeps</u> the urethra closed. It's a bit like a rubber band. Then when you go to the toilet, your brain <u>speaks to</u> the bladder to tighten up and then the urine leaves through the urethra. So you've got all these things <u>working</u> together – bladder, urethra, muscles and nerves and the whole system's got to work. But it doesn't always work efficiently. You can get <u>leaking</u>, you see, caused by your medicines. You have high blood pressure, don't you? Yes, well, medicines to treat high blood pressure sometimes make the sphincter muscles – the ones around the urethra – sometimes they make them too <u>loose</u> and then the urethra doesn't close properly and you get <u>a leak</u>.

There is an obvious remedy – you stop taking the medicines – but in your case I think there may be no alternative – you've got to keep <u>taking</u> them. There are exercises you can do <u>to train</u> your muscles to work better. I can show you these if you like. But don't stop taking the medicine until <u>you've</u> talked to the doctor.

There are other things. Do you drink a lot of coffee? Coffee can <u>give</u> you problems – or chocolate even. Alcohol of course. So you see there are all sorts of causes and no you're not <u>going</u> senile and I know it's <u>embarrassing</u> but this sort of thing affects all sorts of people. You'd be <u>amazed</u> by how many people suffer from it.

And I know there's a stigma <u>attached</u> to incontinence though there's absolutely nothing to be <u>ashamed</u> of. Tell you what, when's your next appointment with your GP? Well, put together a list of all the medicines you <u>take</u> and when you see the doctor ask him if any of them can cause bladder problems and then <u>tell</u> him what you've <u>told</u> me.'

Exercise 16g

1 b.
2 a.
3 c.
4 c. In Scottish English, 'wee' means 'little'.
5 a. Apart from being the excess fat around your stomach, a 'spare tyre' is the extra tyre you keep in the boot of your car.

Exercise 16h

a. 'Brought' has a dual meaning. The nurse means 'what is the reason' or 'why did you come to the hospital?' The patient answers as if 'brought' means 'how?' and 'what transport did you use?'

b. When the clerk calls out 'Mr Wilson's history' he means, 'I've got the file (history) of Mr Wilson'. Mr Wilson interprets the words as 'Mr Wilson <u>is</u> history' meaning 'Mr Wilson is finished' or 'Mr Wilson is going to die'.

c. The sentence literally means that the knee disappeared on the third day. It should say: 'On the second day, the knee was better and on the third day, the wound/bruise/cut/pain, etc. had completely disappeared.'

d. The sentence suggests that the patient is depressed because she is seeing the doctor. It should read something like this: 'I have been seeing the patient ever since her depression started.'

e. The suggestion is that the patient does not have permission to be alive. It should read: 'Discharged himself without permission.'

f. Autopsies are for dead people only. Obviously 'autopsy' is the wrong word.

g. You can commit suicide only once. The sentence should read: '...doesn't have a past history of <u>attempted</u> suicides.'

h. If the patient lay on her left side for over a year, chest pains would be the least of her problems. The sentence should read: 'For over a year the patient has had chest pains when she lies on her left side.'

Chapter Seventeen

Conversations in UK standard English

Conversation 17.1: Nobody told me anything

This is a conversation between a patient and a hospital social worker after the patient had a tracheostomy. The patient speaks in something like 'standard' English. (Adapted from Bridge: *Communication in Nursing Care* Published by Elsevier Science Ltd.)

PATIENT: I couldn't speak at first with the tube down and then I remember the doctor coming over this thing (tracheostomy). But I didn't understand what they were talking about because <u>I never had no trouble with my throat</u> – it was only a bit of bronchitis.

SOCIAL WORKER: Did the tube bother you in your mouth?

PATIENT: Oh yes, and when they put that other big thing on, you know (respirator tubing, etc.) <u>it was *that* heavy</u>.

SOCIAL WORKER: What bothered you about the tube?

PATIENT: Well, it seemed as if it was all wrapped round my gums and my mouth was all swelled, and I've never had cold sores but my lips were sore.

SOCIAL WORKER: How did you feel about it when you couldn't talk? Did it bother you?

PATIENT: Oh yes, I was dead upset, I cried.

SOCIAL WORKER: Did anyone talk to you about it?

PATIENT: No, they (the staff) don't talk much really. No conversation. <u>Don't get me wrong</u>, they do everything they can down there. They're marvellous. When I wanted ice, whatever I wanted, it was there. It was no trouble to them. I never drink tea, only coffee, so if I don't have coffee I'll go all day without a drink. But whatever I wanted, there was no messing about.

SOCIAL WORKER: Did you know what was going on?

PATIENT: Well, I can't say there was anything that bad. Just these tubes in my mouth and my mouth being sore: I mean *if I'd known they were putting them in* it wouldn't have worried me. And I'm trying to take them out so I can explain to them. But I can't. Do you know what I mean? Well, it upset me to think I was just left. I thought I'm going to be a cabbage after all these years of working and thinking about the children. Oh I really did think I wasn't going to get better, I thought well, *rather than suffer and be on their hands I'd rather have gone.*

Exercise 17a

1 When the patient says: 'I never had no trouble with my throat', she means:
a. I've always had trouble with my throat.
b. I've never had trouble with my throat.
c. I don't have trouble with my throat.

2 'it was that heavy' means:
a. it was very heavy.
b. that was heavy.
c. it was not heavy.

3 When the patient says 'don't get me wrong', she is:
a. making a strong complaint.
b. making no complaint.
c. making a mild complaint.

4 'If I'd known they were putting them in' tells us that:
a. the patient worried when she was told about the tracheostomy.
b. the patient knew all about the tracheostomy.
c. the patient was not told anything.

5 When the patient says 'rather than suffer and be on their hands I'd rather have gone' she means:
a. I would have preferred to go to a different hospital.
b. instead of bothering staff it would have been better to leave the hospital.
c. it would have been better to die than to bother the staff.

Conversation 17.2: The gorgeous wash

This is a part of a conversation with a post-operative cardiac patient. She describes how she felt in the days following her operation. (Adapted from Bridge: *Communication in Nursing Care* Published by Elsevier Science Ltd)

You get a sort of feeling you're not sure what day it is, what time it is, what part of the day. It's a most peculiar feeling. You needed to have a bit of reassurance that it's half past eleven on a Saturday morning. Even if you ask that you probably want to ask in half an hour what time it is. You feel awful – but it gives you that reassurance that you know what day it is.

It was worse for me, I wear specs, can't see without them. I left them in the ward. It was about four days before I got them back. I got my specs and I could see the clock and everything, and everything was lovely. Only one as wears specs would understand that – because you don't even hear properly without them.

I don't remember anyone much the first couple of days, but I can remember people saying, 'Susan, we're going to give you a wash' or 'Susan, do that for me', or something or other for me. But mostly it was that gorgeous wash. I don't remember any individual talking to me. But I remember seeing the priest – but he's distinctive.

Exercise 17b

1 When the patient uses the word 'you' she means:
a. herself.
b. the person she is talking to.
c. everyone else.

2 What is 'a most peculiar feeling'?
a. The strangest feeling she has ever had.
b. A very strange feeling.
c. A common feeling.

3 When the patient says 'You feel awful,' she is:
a. sympathising with the person she is talking to.
b. describing how she felt.
c. describing how she feels now.

4 Who is the patient referring to when she says: 'only one as wears specs would understand that'?
a. Another person whom she knows.
b. Any person who wears spectacles.
c. The person she is talking to.

5 What or who are 'them'? ('...you don't even hear properly without them.')
a. Other people who wear spectacles.
b. Hearing aids.
c. Spectacles.

6 'mostly it was that gorgeous wash' refers to:
a. the thing she remembers most clearly.
b. the best thing that happened.
c. the thing that happened most often.

7 Why does she 'remember seeing the priest'?
a. She didn't see anybody else.
b. The priest spoke to her.
c. She could pick him out clearly because of his clothes.

Conversation 17.3: Facing up to death

Mrs Benson has a terminal illness and a nurse visits her at home. At first she is withdrawn and irritable. In the following conversation she tells the nurse that she had been to the hospital on the previous day but she had received no further treatment. This is part of the conversation between Mrs Benson and the nurse. Read it and answer the questions that follow. (Adapted from Bridge: *Communication in Nursing Care* published by Elsevier Science Ltd.)

MRS BENSON [ANGRILY]:   After yesterday, <u>I'm beginning to wonder where all this is going to end</u>. Last time I had this pain, they cured it with treatment, and now <u>they have given me these pills and they're no good at all</u>.

NURSE: It seems that you had a bad day yesterday, Mrs Benson. <u>What exactly happened at the hospital</u>?

MRS BENSON: (near to tears):   Well, <u>to be honest</u> nurse, it started off wrong. I met a lady I often see there and this time she really seemed very ill.

NURSE: That must have been frightening.

MRS BENSON: Yes. She was in such pain and was so weak – I suppose that could happen to me.

[Silence] Nurse tries to show she understands that Mrs Benson is <u>trying to face up to her own deterioration and death</u>.

Exercise 17c

1   When Mrs Benson says: 'I'm beginning to wonder where all this is going to end', she means:
a. I want my illness to end.
b. I don't know when I'm going to get better.
c. I feel confused and frightened.

2   When Mrs Benson says: 'they have given me these pills and they're no good at all', she is expressing:
a. no confidence in the staff at the hospital.
b. disappointment that now there is no hope.
c. a desire for different pills.

3   Why does the nurse ask: 'What exactly happened at the hospital?'
a. To find out more about the pills.
b. Because she needs to know more about what the doctors think.
c. To encourage Mrs Benson to talk.

4   Saying 'to be honest' is a way to:
a. say something she doesn't want to say.
b. say something truthful.
c. emphasise that she is not lying.

5   According to the text, Mrs Benson is 'trying to face up to her own deterioration and death'. This means she is trying:
a. to accept the fact she will not get better.
b. to understand the situation of the lady she knows in the hospital.
c. to fight the illness.

Conversation 17.4: The amputation

This is an account by a man who was in a road accident. He was a passenger in a car in which the driver was killed. (Adapted from a report on the BBC News website 09/01/2002.)

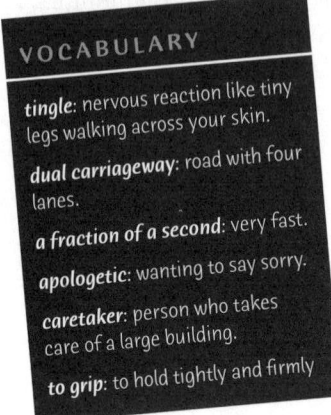

VOCABULARY

tingle: nervous reaction like tiny legs walking across your skin.

dual carriageway: road with four lanes.

a fraction of a second: very fast.

apologetic: wanting to say sorry.

caretaker: person who takes care of a large building.

to grip: to hold tightly and firmly

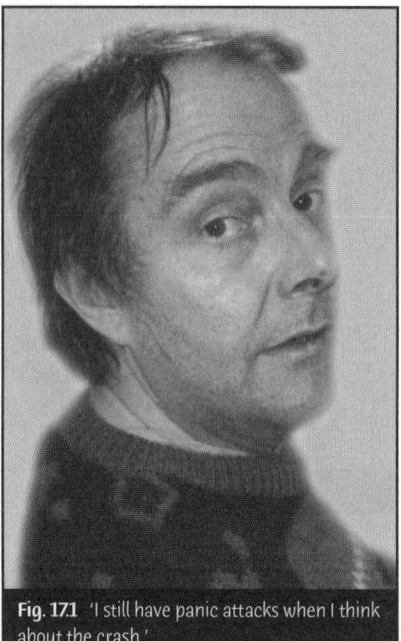

Fig. 17.1 'I still have panic attacks when I think about the crash.'

Sometimes when I talk about the crash I get a panic attack and my breath gets short. Right now I can feel my left hand and fingers start to tingle, even though they're no longer there.

The first and only thing I knew about the actual accident was coming round in the car and seeing my arm hanging off.

It was about ten o'clock and we were driving up the dual carriageway towards our home in Leeds when the other driver come up behind us at 70 mph. He hit us and we went into a lamp-post. We brought it down and that's what took my arm. It all happened in a fraction of a second. A fraction I can't remember. When I came round I was just wondering where I was.

They woke me up in the operating theatre to tell me they were going to amputate my arm at the elbow. After the operation I had to ask which one was missing. I could still feel both.

Whatever happened during the crash, it crushed my elbow and fractured the arm in seven places. It also removed the skin. The surgeon was very apologetic, needlessly, and said it was the only time he'd ever lost an arm.

Just a week after the crash, I asked to leave the hospital bed so I could attend Iris's funeral. I didn't realise it then, but I was in a state of shock that was to last a considerable time.

I later found out he was three times over the limit when he killed my friend and dramatically changed my life forever.

I was a caretaker before the crash and a lot of my work was manual. Even cleaning with one arm is totally impossible, so I had to leave the job and the house that went with it.

I was worse before I was fitted with a prosthetic limb. I'd go to the paper shop and people would immediately <u>clock that I was the wrong shape</u>. Old ladies would hold the door for me. That doesn't happen with the prosthetic arm.

<u>All respect to the NHS</u>, but the arm isn't very good. It's pink, not my skin colour at all, and it causes blisters.

I really want a hand that can grip. I'm hopeful that will end some of the frustration I feel.

As for the man who did this, <u>he doesn't exist. If you hold something against someone that affects you and that's not a part of who I am.</u>

I have to go by the crash site regularly. <u>The new lamp-post really stands out</u> because I can't help looking for it every time.

Exercise 17d

1 His 'breath gets short' because the speaker is:
a. terrified.
b. in great pain.
c. exhausted.

2 'coming round in the car' means:
a. turning to look when he was in the car.
b. becoming conscious.
c. the car was upside down.

3 When the speaker says 'the surgeon was very apologetic, needlessly, and said it was the only time he'd ever lost an arm' he means:
a. the surgeon had no reason to apologise even though he couldn't find the patient's prosthetic arm.
b. the surgeon couldn't save the man's arm, but it wasn't his fault.
c. although this was the first time the surgeon had made a mistake, 'sorry' was just not enough.

4 'to clock I was the wrong shape' means:
a. to always give the wrong time.
b. to see I wasn't like other people.
c. to not understand what I was saying.

5 'All respect to the NHS' means:
a. there is nothing wrong with the NHS.
b. the NHS is no good.
c. the NHS tries its best.

6 When the speaker refers to the man who caused the accident he says: 'He doesn't exist. If you hold something against someone that affects you and that's not part of who I am' he is saying that:
a. he forgives him.
b. he has forgotten him.
c. he hates him.

7 About the crash site, the speaker says 'the new lamp-post really stands out'. From this we understand that:

a. the new lamp-post is different from all the other lamp-posts.

b. the new lamp-post has been put in a new position so that drivers can now see it more clearly.

c. the new lamp-post attracts his attention.

Conversation 17.5: Counselling Roberta

This is the conversation between Roberta Blackwood, the patient who was admitted to hospital after taking an overdose of paracetamol and alcohol (Chapter 5), and a nurse. It takes place some time after Roberta's admission to hospital.

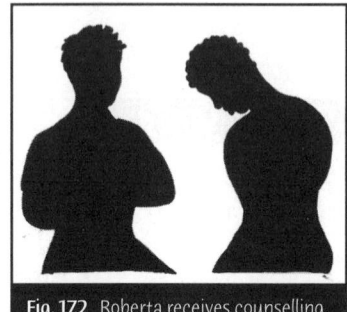

Fig. 17.2 Roberta receives counselling.

NURSE: How you feeling now Roberta? OK?

ROBERTA: OK.

NURSE: <u>You gave us a few scary moments back there</u>.

ROBERTA: Uh huh.

NURSE: You're a daft so and so. What made you do it? Do you want to tell me? Things getting on top of you? Are they? Every little thing?

ROBERTA: S'pose so. Yeah.

NURSE: Look, it's all right. You don't have to tell me anything if you don't want. And if you do, it'll just be between me and you and these four walls. <u>How are things with your chap?</u> Not so good? There. You have a good cry if that's what you want. Here you are, dry your eyes with this.

ROBERTA: Sorry.

NURSE: Don't apologise. You've got nothing to be sorry for. Better out than in, I always think.

ROBERTA [SOBBING]: It's just that it's so bloody hopeless. <u>They'd all be better off without me</u>. They would.

NURSE: Now now. Are you sure that's true?

ROBERTA: Yeah, well, I'm a lousy mother for a start-off. The nipper's always crying. I get so tired. She never stops crying. I can't stop her and she wakes him up and then he starts shouting at me why can't I shut her up? Life's shit. I can't stand it no more.

NURSE: Look, there are people who can help. There are places you can go if you need <u>to get away from it all</u> for a bit. I tell you what. I can talk with the hospital social worker.

ROBERTA: No, not them Social Services.

NURSE: No, not Social Services. Nothing to do with Social Services. I'm talking about Mrs Pugh. She's the lady who was here earlier. Maybe you don't remember. She's lovely, Mrs Pugh. Ever so nice to talk to and she'll <u>be able to sort something out</u> for you and get you some help, I'm sure. Will you let me fix up Mrs Pugh to see you?

Exercise 17e

1 When the nurse says to Roberta, 'You gave us a few scary moments back there,' she means:
a. We were frightened of you.
b. We were worried about you.
c. You were frightened of us.

2 When the nurse asks, 'How are things with your chap?' she wants to know:
a. if her husband is unwell.
b. what her husband is doing.
c. if she is getting on with her husband.

3 When Roberta says 'They'd all be better off without me' she is saying:
a. she costs her family money.
b. it would be good for her family if she died.
c. her life is insured and her family would benefit from her death.

4 'To get away from it all' means:
a. to have a break.
b. to find a solution.
c. to run away.

5 Mrs Pugh will 'be able to sort something out.' In other words, Mrs Pugh will:
a. get help for Roberta.
b. get help with Roberta.
c. get help from Roberta.

Conversation 17.6: Am I dying?

In the following conversation, a nurse talks to a very ill patient who has been brought in to A & E.

NURSE: All right, Mr Ramsbottom? Can you open your eyes? Can you hear me?

MR RAMSBOTTOM: Mmm.

NURSE: Hello. Can you see me now? Don't worry, you're at the hospital. We're taking care of you. Your wife's here too. Everything's going to be all right. Just nod your head if you can hear me. That's good. Well done. We're going to have a good look at your chest. I'm going to ask you some questions as we go along, OK? Important to get some information. Just nod your head. Good. OK. You thought you were having a heart attack, is that right? Right. Did you take anything?

MR RAMSBOTTOM: Aspirin.

NURSE: Aspirin? OK, how many? One? Two? Show me with your fingers.

MR RAMSBOTTOM: Uh.

NURSE: Two. You've had angina? Your wife says. Yes? But never had a heart attack, right? Did your doctor give you any nitroglycerine tablets to take if you had chest pain? Yes?

MR RAMSBOTTOM: Couldn't find them. I dunno where. Maybe run out. But it can't be. Haven't used them all.

NURSE: But no pain now? All clear at the moment? Right. Well you did the right thing phoning 999. I don't think you're having a heart attack, Mr Ramsbottom, but we'll make sure everything's <u>hunky dory</u>. What we're going to do is, we're going to give you an ECG. Do you know what that is? It's a tracing of your heart – it'll tell us what's going on – give us a picture.

NURSE: So what were you doing when you had the pain?

MR RAMSBOTTOM: Oh, just <u>poking around in the garden</u> doing <u>odd jobs</u> and that. Some bending over but nothing heavy.

NURSE: I see.

MR RAMSBOTTOM: And <u>I couldn't put me hands on the nitro</u>.

NURSE: Uh huh.

MR RAMSBOTTOM: It started in the left-hand side of me chest and spread. Up here.

NURSE: It's all right. Don't move, lie as still as you can.

MR RAMSBOTTOM: And I couldn't breathe. Sweating like a pig I was. Nurse, am I having a heart attack? Nurse?

NURSE: Here's the doctor, he's going to take over now.

Exercise 17f   **Which of the following statements are grammatically correct?**

a. Mr Ramsbottom hasn't have a heart attack.
b. Mr Ramsbottom hasn't had a heart attack.
c. Mr Ramsbottom has angina.
d. Mr Ramsbottom have angina.
e. Mr Ramsbottom gets angina.
f. Mr Ramsbottom ran out of nitroglycerine.
g. Mr Ramsbottom ran out in nitroglycerine.
h. The nurse asks the patient he has a tracing of his heart.
i. The nurse tells the patient he is going to make a tracing of his heart.
j. Mr Ramsbottom fears of dying.
k. Mr Ramsbottom is afraid of dying.
l. Information comes the patient's wife.
m. Information is from the patient's wife.

Exercise 17g

1   The gesture which means 'yes' is a nod of the head. What means 'no'?
a. a twist of the head.
b. a shake of the head.
c. a turn of the head.

2   If a nurse asks a patient 'Do you take anything?' the nurse means:
a. 'Have you brought anything with you?'
b. 'Do you want medicine?'
c. 'Do you use any medicine?'

3 When something is 'hunky dory' it is:
a. going wrong.
b. fine.
c. not looking good.

4 Doing 'odd jobs' is doing:
a. strange and unusual things.
b. secret and hidden things.
c. small things.

5 When the patient says he has been 'poking around in the garden' he means he has been:
a. doing this and that.
b. digging.
c. resting.

6 The patient couldn't put his hands on the nitro. This means:
a. he dropped the nitro.
b. he couldn't find the nitro.
c. he couldn't reach the nitro.

Conversation 17.7: Problems with mother

The following conversation is between a nurse and the relatives of an elderly woman who lives with them. They are telling the nurse how difficult it is to care for the old lady.

NURSE: So, things are getting a bit difficult at home?

MR DOBBS: That's an understatement, nurse.

NURSE: Mmm. I suppose you were warned about what might happen with your mother?

MRS DOBBS: But you never know until it hits you, do you? I mean, poor thing – sometimes she's quite doolally and sometimes right as rain. She can flip just like that and the lapses can come on quite out of the blue.

VOCABULARY

understatement: something that is true but deliberately doesn't express how serious things are.

doolally: mad.

lapse: failure/decline in condition.

out of the blue: suddenly and unexpectedly.

gone out: absent-minded/blank.

yo-yo: toy that goes up and down on a string.

patchy: not consistent.

kid sister: younger sister.

say: for example.

woolly: cardigan/jumper.

to fumble: to have awkward use of fingers.

dribble: uncontrolled saliva.

to see things: to hallucinate/see things which other people do not see.

compos mentis: having a proper grasp on reality.

to sit bolt upright: sit stiffly and alertly.

nineteen to the dozen: a lot.

NURSE: And...?

MRS DOBBS: Sometimes it can be quite funny really, but mostly it's horrible. I mean she forgets everything and gets it all mixed up. I mean she used to be so independent. You know – she used to do everything for herself. And now look! I'm sure it's terrible for her. Worse for her than it is for us.

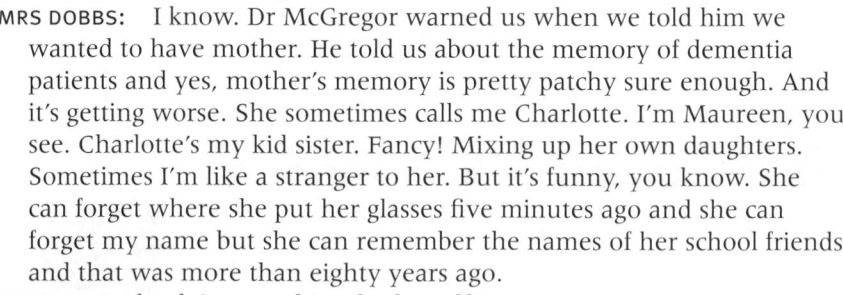

Fig. 173 Mrs Dobbs' mother stabs herself because she can't see clearly.

MR DOBBS: When she's at her worst she's really gone out, if you know what I mean. Night-time! Cor! Your mother's up and down like a yo-yo all night some nights, isn't she?

NURSE: Yes, you can expect that.

MRS DOBBS: I know. Dr McGregor warned us when we told him we wanted to have mother. He told us about the memory of dementia patients and yes, mother's memory is pretty patchy sure enough. And it's getting worse. She sometimes calls me Charlotte. I'm Maureen, you see. Charlotte's my kid sister. Fancy! Mixing up her own daughters. Sometimes I'm like a stranger to her. But it's funny, you know. She can forget where she put her glasses five minutes ago and she can forget my name but she can remember the names of her school friends and that was more than eighty years ago.

NURSE: Is she doing anything for herself?

MRS DOBBS: Less and less these days. Most days she's OK about getting dressed, say, but like yesterday she couldn't control her fingers and it was heart-breaking to see her fumbling about with the buttons on her woolly.

NURSE: Eating?

MR DOBBS: Oh, I don't mind if she needs a hand sometimes, it's just that she's proud and wants to do stuff herself. Doesn't want fuss, you know.

MRS DOBBS: She's slow, just needs time. Really she's very good. She really tries. She's a bit of a dribbler! [laughs] Sorry. I mean she can make a bit of a mess, bless her! She can miss the plate entirely. Yesterday she stabbed herself with her fork.

NURSE: It might be that she's having trouble with her eyes as well. Maybe she can't see the food clearly or she's seeing double. You could try using a plain plate, put the food on a plain plate and she will see it better.

MR DOBBS: OK. Good idea. We'll try that. You know she sees things too. Don't know how much, she won't always say. People mostly, and voices of people she knew in the past, childhood even. She tells me about it, you know, when she's compos mentis. That's how I know.

NURSE: Yes, a lot of people say this. But this hallucinating – it's not frightening her is it?

MRS DOBBS: No, the other day she was sitting bolt upright in bed chatting to someone. Chatting cheerfully away nineteen to the dozen with George and he's been dead some ten years now. But for her, you know, he was there. Really there. But afterwards she knows he can't have been there. She's quite rational sometimes.

NURSE: Any constipation?

MRS DOBBS: It's the drugs, I think.

NURSE: Yes, quite possible. They can cause dehydration. If it's a problem we can always have a look at the possibility of changing her medication.

Exercise 17h

Answer the following questions by choosing an answer from a, b and c:

1   Mrs Dobbs says her mother can 'flip'. This means she:
a. changes quickly.
b. can fall over at any time.
c. can be physically violent.

2   'Mother's memory is pretty patchy' means that mother.
a. forgets everything.
b. forgets nothing.
c. forgets a lot.

3   Mother 'needs a hand' means that she:
a. requires assistance.
b. is independent.
c. cannot hold things.

4   The nurse thinks that perhaps Mrs Dobbs's mother stabbed herself because:
a. she is unco-ordinated.
b. she is co-ordinated.
c. she has good co-ordination.

5   'Chatting away to George nineteen to the dozen' means that she was:
a. talking rapidly about numbers with George.
b. talking intensely about George.
c. having an involved conversation with George.

Exercise 17i

After this conversation the nurse makes the following record of what she has learnt from Mr and Mrs Dobbs. Complete the report by choosing the correct word from each of the brackets:

Patient's relatives experiencing some difficulties. Patient (have, has, had) patchy memory and (mixes, mix, mixed) up daughters and forgets their names. Patient showing (decrease, decreasing, to decrease) ability (to cope, cope, coped) with ADLs – unco-ordinated – cannot (done up, doing up, do up) buttons and has problems (to control, control over, controlling) knife and fork. Vision probably (decay, decays, decaying) rapidly. Relatives report patient has visual and auditory (hallucinating, hallucinate, hallucinations). Patient (constipation, has constipated, constipated).

Conversation 17.8: What will tomorrow bring?

This is a conversation that takes place late at night on a hospital ward. The patient is going to have an operation in the morning and speaks to a nurse.

MRS BROWN: I don't want to make a big song and dance about this, nurse, but I'm absolutely parched. Do you think I could have something to wet my whistle?

NURSE: Let's have a look at your notes. Oh, I'm sorry, Barbara. 'Nil by mouth' is what it says here. You're in theatre in the morning.

MRS BROWN: My lips are all dry and cracked. Listen to me! Sound like a frog.

NURSE: I tell you what, I'll give you something to swill round in your mouth. Don't swallow though.

MRS BROWN: Thanks.

NURSE: Here you go. That's it, just enough to keep your mouth moist. Spit into this. Good. How's that? Any better?

MRS BROWN: Thanks nurse.

NURSE: Can't you sleep?

MRS BROWN: No. Too bloody nervous. Excuse my French.

NURSE: There's nothing to worry about, Barbara. The surgeon's very good, you know. He's done loads of these. He can do them blindfold. Really, you'll be fine. It'll be over in a jiffy and you'll be in and out like a dose of salts.

MRS BROWN: All right.

NURSE: You met him yesterday, didn't you? The surgeon?

MRS BROWN: The tall man? Bow tie. Bald as a coot he is. That one?

NURSE: That's him.

MRS BROWN: Nice chap. Nice hands. I remember his spotless hands. He called me his 'pet'. Wasn't that nice?

NURSE: Yes. So you can trust him to do a good job.

MRS BROWN: Right, but...

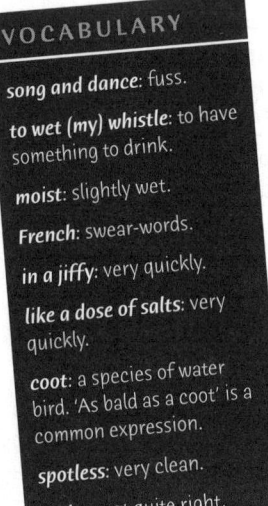

VOCABULARY

song and dance: fuss.

to wet (my) whistle: to have something to drink.

moist: slightly wet.

French: swear-words.

in a jiffy: very quickly.

like a dose of salts: very quickly.

coot: a species of water bird. 'As bald as a coot' is a common expression.

spotless: very clean.

dodgy: not quite right.

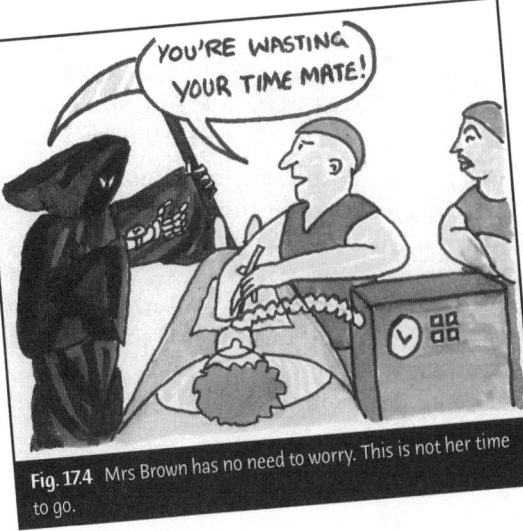

Fig. 17.4 Mrs Brown has no need to worry. This is not her time to go.

NURSE: 'But' what?

MRS BROWN: People die, don't they? I mean, they can die under the knife. I'm a bit frightened. I don't mind admitting it. But I suppose if it's my time to go, it's my time to go.

NURSE: Well yes, I suppose so. There is always a risk, but I've got a good feeling about this one. About you. And my intuition's never wrong. Never.

MRS BROWN: Do you think so? I hope you're right, but you know, I've got a dodgy feeling about it. It's just a feeling, but you know…

NURSE: Everything'll be fine. You just see. We've all got our fingers crossed for you, but you won't need it – everything'll be right as rain. Tomorrow night you'll sleep like a log and on Thursday we'll look back on this and have a good old laugh about it, you and me. OK?

Exercise 17j

Here are some questions about the conversation you have just read. Choose the correct answer from a, b and c:

1 What does the nurse refuse to give Barbara?
a. A drink.
b. Something to eat.
c. A sedative to help her sleep.

2 The nurse gives Barbara something for her dry mouth but what does she tell her to do?
a. Gargle.
b. Drink slowly.
c. Rinse her mouth.

3 When the patient refers to her 'time to go' she is talking about:
a. the time of the operation.
b. dying.
c. how long she must wait.

4 The nurse tells Mrs Brown that the surgeon is:
a. experienced.
b. meticulous.
c. well qualified.

5 What is happening if you are 'under the knife'?
a. You are dead.
b. You are being attacked.
c. You are undergoing surgery.

6 When the nurse says she has a 'good feeling' she means:
a. she is feeling happy.
b. she is feeling positive.
c. she is feeling well.

Exercise 17k

Take idioms from the conversation you have just read and use them to replace the expressions in brackets in the following sentences.

1 The Staff Nurse made a (big thing) out of my little mistake.

2 The patient's throat is dry and he says he (could murder a cup of tea).

3 I was in and out of the doctor's surgery (in the wink of an eye).

4 I know this job so well, I could do it (backwards).

5 You've got a (dicky) heart and you must be careful what you do.

Answers and comments on the language

Exercise 17a

1 b. Here is the double negative again (see Exercise 15b, Question 2).

2 a. 'That' can mean 'very' or 'a lot'. For example,'He had that much pain' means 'He had a lot of pain.' 'She was that unhappy at home' means 'She was very unhappy at home.'

3 c. This is an example of 'down-playing'. The patient wants to complain but is rather reserved about doing so. She is saying 'I am grateful for everything they've done, BUT...'

4 c. The patient is complaining that medical staff did not communicate anything to her. She is saying that if someone had spoken to her about what they were doing instead of treating her like an object then she wouldn't have felt so bad.

5 c. The patient feels she has been treated very badly and disrespectfully and she is actually very angry. This final comment is a way of saying that the medical staff made her feel as if she was a nuisance. Her comment about dying is the desperate expression of someone who feels that death is the only act of control over the situation she has left, and in a way it would teach everyone a lesson if she died.

Exercise 17b

1 a. 'You' often means 'I' in speech, especially when someone (like this patient) is trying to describe an experience which is both personal and also common to a lot of people.

2 b. 'Most' here means 'very'. It is often used to give strong emphasis. 'It was a most unhappy time' means 'it was a very unhappy time'. Compare this with 'it was <u>the</u> most unhappy time (of my life)' which would mean there has never been a more unhappy time.

3 b. 'You' is the speaker (me/I). 'Feel' means 'felt'. Very often a story is told in the present tense even though the events were in the past. For example: 'There's this man and he's walking down the road when he sees a dog...'

4 b. 'as' here means 'who'.

5 c. Spectacles are grammatically plural.

6 b. This sentence describes a very pleasant memory in a lot of unpleasant memories. 'It' refers to the best thing she remembers.

7 c. She says that the priest is 'distinctive'. She cannot see properly because she hasn't got her glasses so out of all the misty shapes in front of her eyes, she was able to distinguish the priest because of his black clothes.

Exercise 17c

1   c. 'I don't know where it will all end' expresses anxiety about the future. Deep down, Mrs Benson knows she is going to die but at the moment she can't make this knowledge conscious – or at least can't get herself to say it.

2   b. Everything Mrs Benson says betrays her terrible fears. Her anger is covering up her fears and she is blaming everything else – her treatment in particular.

3   c. An open-ended question like the one the nurse asks is a device to get the patient to talk so that she can 'let it all out'.

4   a. Seeing the lady at the hospital upset Mrs Benson badly and 'to be honest' is a device used to introduce something which she is half-reluctant to confront. In this case it is the fact that the lady at the hospital is a reflection of herself and her own situation.

5   a. 'To face up to' something is to accept something unpleasant or difficult.

Exercise 17d

1   a. The speaker uses 'gets' with 'short' to mean 'becomes'.

2   b. 'To come round' is to regain consciousness or to wake up. The *speaker* 'comes round', not the car (options **a** and **c**).

3   b. The surgeon 'loses the man's arm', means that the surgeon cannot save the man's arm and has to amputate. Note that, although the arm belongs to the speaker, both he and the surgeon refer to the arm as if it belongs to the surgeon. Not only do people 'lose' limbs, they also 'lose' their lives when they die.

4   b. 'To clock someone or something' is a fairly common English colloquialism which means 'to see' or 'to recognise'. It has nothing to do with clocks or time (option **a**).

5   c. The speaker is making a mild complaint. He is saying first that he appreciates all that the NHS does BUT...

6   a. 'To hold something against someone' is to hold a grudge or stay angry with someone for doing you some harm. The speaker is trying hard to not hold anything against the man who caused the crash. When the speaker says 'He doesn't exist' it suggests that he tries hard not to think about the man who caused the crash. In the second sentence, he amends this to say that he doesn't think badly about the man.

7   c. 'To stand out' usually means to look or to be different from things around. However, in this case the speaker can't stop himself from looking for that one particular lamp-post. So he is saying that the fact it looks different is really only in his mind.

Exercise 17e

1   b. 'Scary' is an adjective from 'scare'. 'We were worried about you' means that we were concerned for your safety.

2   c. 'To get on with someone' is to have a good relationship with them.

3   b. It is true that to be 'well off' and to be 'better off' refer to having money and wealth but, in the context of her suicide attempt, Roberta is referring to something more general. She is saying they would feel happier if she died.

4   a. 'To get away from it all' is an expression often used to advertise holidays. 'It' is the stresses and strains of everyday life which you temporarily leave behind. 'To run away' is to escape, probably permanently.

5   a. 'To get help <u>with</u> Roberta' (option **b**) suggests that Roberta is a problem for Mrs Pugh and that she now needs help dealing with Roberta.

Exercise 17f

The following statements are grammatically correct:

b.

c.

e. There is often no difference between 'has angina' and 'gets angina' though 'gets angina' does suggest that he has attacks of angina that come and go.

f.

i.

k.

m.

Exercise 17g

1   b.

2   c.

3   b.

4   c. 'Odd' sometimes means 'strange'. An 'odd' number is any number that cannot be divided by 2. However, 'odd jobs' are things like minor repairs.

5   a. To 'poke around' in this context means to do nothing in particular – the same as to do 'this and that'.

6   b.

Exercise 17h

1   a. 'To flip' can mean 'to quickly turn over', for example, to flip a page or to flip a coin. Generally it means to change from one thing to its opposite – up to down, happy to sad, etc.

2 c. A 'patch' can be a piece of material covering a hole, for example on a pair of trousers or the inner tube of a tyre. It can also mean 'a small area', for example 'a patch of grass'.

3 a. If someone needs help, you 'lend a hand' or 'give a hand'.

4 a.

5 c. An 'involved' conversation is an 'intense' or 'deep' conversation.

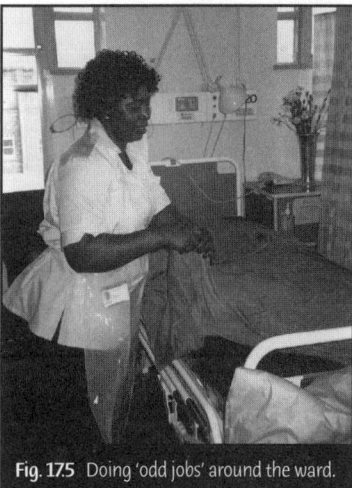

Fig. 17.5 Doing 'odd jobs' around the ward.

Exercise 17i

Patient's relatives experiencing some difficulties. Patient <u>has</u> patchy memory and <u>mixes</u> up daughters and forgets their names. Patient showing <u>decreasing</u> ability <u>to cope</u> with ADLs – unco-ordinated – cannot <u>do up</u> buttons and has problems <u>controlling</u> knife and fork. Vision probably <u>decaying</u> rapidly. Relatives report patient has visual and auditory <u>hallucinations</u>. Patient <u>constipated</u>.

Exercise 17j

1 a.

2 c. 'To gargle' (option **a**) is what you do with an antiseptic for a sore throat.

3 b. There are lots of euphemisms for dying and death. See 'Medical euphemisms' in Chapter 16.

4 a.

5 c.

6 b. 'To have a good feeling' here is different in meaning from 'feeling good', which usually means 'feeling happy'.

Exercise 17k

1 The staff nurse made a <u>song and dance</u> about my little mistake.

2 The patient's throat is dry and he needs <u>to wet his whistle</u>. He says he could murder a cup of tea. (Note that 'could murder' here means 'to want', for example, 'I could murder a cigarette.')

3 I was in and out of the doctor's surgery <u>in a jiffy</u>/<u>like a dose of salts</u>.

4 I know this job so well I could do it <u>blindfold</u>.

5 You've got a <u>dodgy</u> heart and you must be careful what you do.

Chapter Eighteen

Conversations in UK regional dialects

Conversation 18.1: The dangerous cucumber

This conversation is between a nurse and a patient who has had an accident at home. The patient speaks with a northern English dialect (Lancashire/Yorkshire).

NURSE: I've got a short accident report to fill in here, Mr Parker. Hope you don't mind a few questions?

MR PARKER: No, you're all right nurse. Fire away.

NURSE: So. The accident … Domestic? Highway? Workplace? In your home, wasn't it? So … Domestic. I'll tick that.

MR PARKER: Aye. In t'kitchen.

NURSE: Right you are. I'll tick this box. 'Kitchen'. What. Fall over, did you?

MR PARKER: Well, aye, in a manner of speaking, happen I did.

NURSE: So what caused the accident? What gave you the cut on the head?

MR PARKER: It were cucumber that done it.

NURSE: A cucumber? That's a new one on me. I never heard of someone being attacked by a cucumber. Dangerous cucumber was it, Mr Parker?

MR PARKER: Give over, nurse. I swear. It were a cucumber.

NURSE: Get away!

MR PARKER: I were helping me missus out, like. 'Slice this' she says. 'And mind yer fingers yer daft ha'p'orth.' So I'm cutting this cucumber up right nice and door flies open and nipper bursts in running like a bat out of hell and yelling at top of her lungs. 'What's all t' fuss?' I shouts, but it were too late and her comes belting straight into us. Up goes cucumber and knife and when I bends over to pick 'em up like, I only goes and forgets cupboard door over me head. Gets up. Bang. Out like a light. Next thing I knows I'm in ruddy ambulance teararsin' down t'street, lights, siren, t' works.

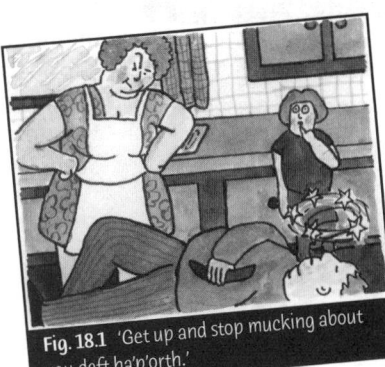

Fig. 18.1 'Get up and stop mucking about you daft ha'p'orth.'

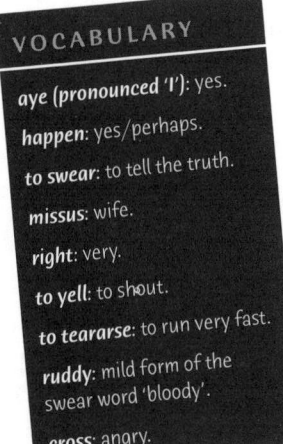

VOCABULARY

aye (pronounced 'I'): yes.

happen: yes/perhaps.

to swear: to tell the truth.

missus: wife.

right: very.

to yell: to shout.

to teararse: to run very fast.

ruddy: mild form of the swear word 'bloody'.

cross: angry.

MRS PARKER: That's right, nurse. He dropped t'ground like a stone. I thought he were just kidding and I were going to give him a piece of my mind, I can tell you. But I sees he's gone white as a ghost. 'Get up' I says. Cross, like. 'Get up and stop mucking about'.

Exercise 18a

Which three of the following idioms mean 'I am joking'?

a. I'm a bat out of hell.
b. I'm having you on.
c. I'm out like a light.
d. I'm a daft ha'p'orth.
e. I'm kidding you.
f. I'm mucking about.
g. I'm making a fuss.

Exercise 18b

Choose the best meaning from a, b and c of the following idioms which are used in the conversation you have just read:

1   'No, you're all right.'
a. I can't.
b. Yes, I can.
c. Don't ask me.

2   'Fire away'.
a. Stand clear.
b. Go ahead.
c. Do it quickly.

3   'Give over'.
a. I mean it.
b. Stop doing that.
c. Listen to me.

4   'Daft ha'p'orth.'
a. Loveable fool.
b. Madman.
c. Useless man.

5   'Nipper'.
a. Dog.
b. Child.
c. Mother.

6   'Belting'.
a. Kicking.
b. Being quiet.
c. Running fast.

7   To go 'out like a light'.
a. To leave the room.
b. To become unconscious.
c. To fall down.

8 'The works'.
   a. Mechanical parts.
   b. A factory.
   c. Everything.

9 To 'give a piece of my mind' (to someone).
   a. to tell off.
   b. to share a thought.
   c. to help.

Conversation 18.2: A fuss about nothing

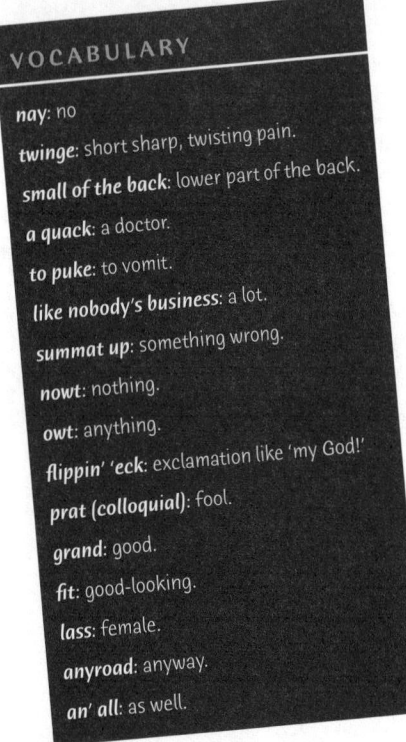

VOCABULARY

nay: no

twinge: short sharp, twisting pain.

small of the back: lower part of the back.

a quack: a doctor.

to puke: to vomit.

like nobody's business: a lot.

summat up: something wrong.

nowt: nothing.

owt: anything.

flippin' 'eck: exclamation like 'my God!'

prat (colloquial): fool.

grand: good.

fit: good-looking.

lass: female.

anyroad: anyway.

an' all: as well.

The next speaker also uses a northern English dialect.

It were last Thursday – nay – it were Friday. I got this twinge. Just here it were, in t'small of me back, and feeling like I wants to puke all the time. Me back hurt like nobody's business. And I thought, 'flippin' 'eck, there must be summat up!' I were a bit frit, you know. At my age like, you've got to watch out for owt and get advice.

So I goes down t' medical centre. Felt like a bit of a prat like – making a fuss about nowt – but I reckoned it were best thing to do.

Did you know that the new quack's a lass? She's a grand lass, aye, fit an' all. I wish I were a few years younger. But all respect to her, she knows her job. Anyroad, she has a good gander and tells me it's owt about nowt, but I were right to come she says. So I'm not fussed about it no more. Still hurts though. But I don't reckon I'll be pushing up daisies for a fair bit yet.'

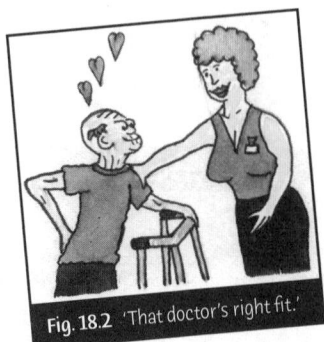

Fig. 18.2 'That doctor's right fit.'

Exercise 18c

Replace the northern English dialect in the sentences that follow with either a, b or c (standard English) so that the meanings of the sentences don't change.

1 We thought there must be (summat up) when he started coughing up blood.
   a. a problem
   b. nothing wrong
   c. anything wrong

2 Look out for (owt) and tell the doctor if you're worried.
   a. something
   b. anything
   c. everything

3 Those nurses are (grand lasses) and all respect to them.
   a. good-looking girls
   b. big women
   c. fine women

4 That doctor's (right fit).
   a. a good one.
   b. very strong.
   c. very handsome.

5 Take off your shirt and I'll (have a gander at) your chest.
   a. listen carefully to
   b. do a thorough examination of
   c. give you some treatment for

6 Frankly, I think it's (owt about nowt) and I'm not going to get worried.
   a. nothing important
   b. very serious
   c. an unnecessary fuss

7 The surgeon asked me if I wanted general or local anaesthetic but I wasn't (fussed) about it.
   a. bothered
   b. amused
   c. scared

Exercise 18d   This is a collection of English idioms used in connection with medicine:

VOCABULARY

to be at death's door: to be close to dying.

to be back on (your) feet: to be healthy again.

to break out: to suddenly have a rash or skin disorder.

to breathe (your) last: to die.

to come round: to regain consciousness.

to catch your death of cold: to get a bad cold/flu.

to feel on top of the world: to feel healthy and happy.

to flare up: to get suddenly worse.

to look the picture of health: to look very healthy.

to run a temperature: to have a high temperature.

to get/become run down: get into poor physical condition.

to throw up: to vomit.

to be under the weather: not feeling well.

Choose an idiom from a, b and c to replace the words in brackets in the following sentences:

1 The ambulance crew found the driver (in mortal danger).
   a. under the weather.
   b. breaking out.
   c. at death's door.

2 He stayed out all night in the rain and (got ill).
   a. caught his death of cold.
   b. breathed his last.
   c. got run down.

3 Overwork and poor diet caused him to (become unhealthy).
   a. run a temperature.
   b. throw up.
   c. become run down.

4 The patient complained of stomach pains and was (being sick) every few minutes.
   a. throwing up
   b. flaring up
   c. coming round

5 On Saturday night he lost consciousness but he didn't (die) until Monday morning.
   a. breathe his last
   b. look the picture of health
   c. catch his death of cold

6 The child (has) a high temperature and needs to be watched very closely.
   a. is running
   b. is flaring up
   c. has broken out

7 Mrs Brown's skin problems (get worse) when she uses scented soap.
   a. become run down
   b. come round
   c. flare up

Conversation 18.3: Mrs Patel's family worries

This is a conversation between a nurse and a patient in hospital. The patient is worried about her son. She speaks with a West Midlands (Birmingham) dialect.

VOCABULARY

to get on me wick: get on my nerves, to be annoying.

girrus: give me.

to cop hold: to take.

safta: this afternoon.

tennarf (doesn't half): a lot.

to pong: to smell.

bab/duck: endearments for both men and women.

loo: toilet.

our bab: youngest child in a family.

ta: thank you.

to wag it: to play truant from school.

to blart on: complain and make a fuss.

GCSEs: UK national examinations.

the dole: unemployment benefit.

to give gob: to be cheeky/answer back/be abusive.

lard 'ed: (lard head) fool.

horse pickle: hospital.

or roight: alright.

mucker: best friend.

bostin: good, great.

NURSE: How you doing, Mrs Patel?

MRS PATEL: Or roight bab.

NURSE: What about the pain? How is it?

MRS PATEL: Hurts something terrible and it's really getting on me wick. Can't you girrus something for it?

NURSE: Oh dear. Same place?

MRS PATEL: No, all over. No kidding, feel like I wanna scream sometimes.

NURSE: Yes. When did we last give you something for it? Let's have a look at the notes. Yes. It's probably time now. Here you are. Swallow these two pills. Here you are, drink this. Swallow. OK?

MRS PATEL: Ta. Here y'ar'. Finished. Cop hold o' this, duck.

NURSE: Right, I'll just put it over here. Have you had your shower?

MRS PATEL: Yeah I had one safta. Don't like that disinfectant though. Tennarf pong.

NURSE: Yes.

MRS PATEL: And me ankles hurt an' all. Look at them. All puffed up and swollen. Can't hardly walk. It were difficult earlier getting to the loo.

NURSE: Did you get there by yourself in the end?

MRS PATEL: I suppose so. I don't want to cause no trouble like. It takes me a long time hobbling all the way down there but I don't want to cause no trouble for no one.

NURSE: Well done, Mrs Patel. We are a bit pushed at the moment and anything you can do for yourself will help. But only if you can.

MRS PATEL: Ta, duck.

NURSE: And will you see Mr Patel today? Will he be coming over?

MRS PATEL: He come over and brung me them flowers. Ain't that sweet?

NURSE: Lovely, dear. Everything OK at home?

MRS PATEL: Or roight, I suppose. Our bab's in trouble at school again. I don't know! My hubby says he's been wagging it every day this week and yesterday he got caught in New Street and now there's all sorts of palaver about it with the school and that. There's his teacher blartin' on about missing them GCSEs. I don't know. If he's not careful he'll end up on the dole – or worse. He's a real handful at the moment is our bab. Tell him anything and he just gives you gob. Probably something to do with me being in here. It's upset him like and he don't get enough attention from his dad – great lard 'ed. The sooner I get out of this horse pickle and back home, the better for everyone.

NURSE: I see. Have you got anyone else who can help out at home? I mean when you go home you'll need to stay in bed a while and take it easy for at least a fortnight.

MRS PATEL: Well, me neighbours are good to me and I've got me mucker – Eileen. They'll all give me a hand with shopping an' that.

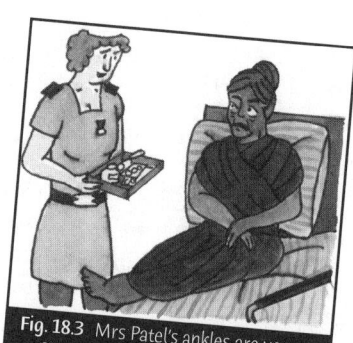

Fig. 18.3 Mrs Patel's ankles are very puffy and swollen but at the moment they're the least of her worries.

NURSE: You'll have to get your kids to help you.

MRS PATEL: Them! Can't get them off their behinds and from out in front of the telly. And they've got their Play Station. They can sit for hours with that blastid thing.

NURSE: You ought to switch it off and tell them you'll throw it away if they don't lend a hand.

MRS PATEL: I suppose so.

NURSE: How does it feel now? The pain I mean?

MRS PATEL: Better – I can feel it fading off. Bostin them pills, ain't they?

Exercise 18e

1   When Mrs Patel asks for something to kill the pain the nurse says 'it's probably time now'. What does she mean?
a. This is a good time.
b. There is plenty of time.
c. This is the correct scheduled time.

2   The nurses are 'a bit pushed at the moment'. This means:
a. short of staff and with too much work to do.
b. getting plenty of free time right now.
c. over-staffed.

3   When the nurse says that Mrs Patel, should make her children 'lend a hand' she is suggesting that:
a. the children should keep out of the way.
b. they should help out with the chores.
c. they should give or loan their mother some money.

4   When Mrs Patel says 'cop hold o' this' she is:
a. taking something from the nurse.
b. giving something to the nurse.
c. asking for something from the nurse.

5   According to Mrs Patel, her husband 'come over and brung me them flowers'. This means:
a. her husband will be coming later and bringing flowers.
b. her husband has come and brought some flowers.
c. her husband came earlier, brought flowers and he has now gone.

6   Mrs Patel has a problem with her youngest child. He is:
a. leaving school.
b. out of work.
c. not going to school.

7   She is afraid her 'bab' will 'end up on the dole'. In other words she is worried that:
a. her son will lose his job.
b. her son will qualify for unemployment benefit.
c. her son will not be qualified for a job.

8   Mrs Patel can't get her children 'off their behinds'. This means her children:
a. are behind with their schoolwork.
b. are disabled and can't move.
c. are lazy.

Exercise 18f

Which of the following statements are true?

a. Mrs Patel is getting on the nurse's nerves.
b. The disinfectant is smelly.
c. Mrs Patel can't get to the toilet by herself.
d. Mrs Patel has an only child.
e. Mrs Patel's son is rude to his mother.
f. Mrs Patel must rest at home for two weeks.
g. Mrs Patel gets a hand from friends.
h. Mrs Patel likes computer games.
i. The nurse advises Mrs Patel to threaten her children.
j. The painkillers work.

Conversation 18.4: The Bugs Bunny episode

VOCABULARY

that ain't the half of it: that's an understatement.

right: very.

to get it: understand.

up West: to the city centre of London.

glad rags: best clothes.

Home Counties: region around London.

to be cream crackered: to rhyme with 'knackered' meaning tired.

to Adam and Eve: to believe.

Uncle Ted: bed.

jam jar: car.

china: china plate = mate/friend.

gear: clothes.

two-and-eight: state/upset.

Bugs Bunny: money.

clobber: clothes.

give us a bell: phone me.

The next conversation is between a nurse and a patient who has been admitted to hospital. The patient is from London and speaks using a cockney dialect.

NURSE: You've been feeling poorly?

JOHN CLARKE: Blimey, that ain't the half of it.

NURSE: What happened? Hypoglycaemia? Did you have an insulin reaction? An episode?

JOHN CLARKE: Yeah. Hypoglycaemia. I'd like, been Jimmy Hill all day – I was irritable…

NURSE: Jimmy Hill?

JOHN CLARKE: That's cockney rhyming slang that is – Jimmy Hill – ill. Get it? Anyway, I was irritable and that. Snapping people's heads off – a right grumpy git. Anyway, me and the missus was going up West. She was in her glad rags – all done up like a dog's dinner and me in me whistle.

NURSE: Sorry?

JOHN CLARKE: Whistle. Whistle and flute – suit. You're not from round here are you?

NURSE: No. Home Counties, me.

JOHN CLARKE: Like I says, I was absolutely cream crackered. Talk about feeling Hank Marvin.

NURSE: Hank Marvin – starvin'. Right? You were hungry. I'm getting the hang of this.

JOHN CLARKE: That's the ticket, darling. And then I goes blank and the next thing, would you Adam and Eve it? I'm lying in this hospital – all tucked up nice and cosy in this here Uncle Ted. Hospital! Blimey! Imagine if I'd blacked out driving the old jam jar! Gave me a hell of a shock I can tell you.

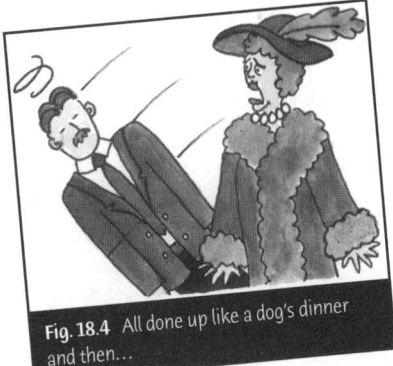

Fig. 18.4 All done up like a dog's dinner and then…

NURSE: Yes. Very tricky. Do you know what caused the episode?

JOHN CLARKE: Well, it was me blood sugar level, weren't it?

NURSE: Mmm. Certainly sounds like it. It can happen very quickly. Somebody's told you about always carrying something with you to eat, haven't they? Something with sugar in it?

JOHN CLARKE: Yeah. Oh yeah. Well nurse, I forgot. That's the plain truth. It just slipped me mind. You see me and me china have just started this little business, haven't we? And yesterday we had this little number on didn't we? Well we had to shift two thousand pairs of Lesley Crowthers. Lesley Crowthers – trousers. And twice as many Eddie Grundies.

NURSE: Let me do it. Eddie Grundies – undies. Right?

JOHN CLARKE: Nice one. All best quality gear. And we'd been running about like blue-arsed flies all day. I was in a right two-and-eight in case we ran out of time – I mean, we're talking big Bugs Bunny here. And we had to be all done by nine. So, I forgot didn't I? It's all right darling, it won't happen again, my missus'll see to that.

NURSE: And you'll measure your blood glucose regularly?

JOHN CLARKE: Yeah. Straight up, love. I ain't going through that again. I've got a meter now and I'll watch it very careful. Don't worry about that.

NURSE: Good. So, is there anything else? Got any questions?

JOHN CLARKE: Only one. Do you or any of the other nurses need any nice clobber? You know, very best merchandise.

NURSE: Well, I don't know…

JOHN CLARKE: Yeah, well, here's me business card. There's me mobile number, give us a bell if you need anything and I'll give you a special price. OK? Don't forget now.

Exercise 18g   **Complete the following report on this patient by choosing the correct verb form from the brackets:**

Mr John Clarke .... (suffering, suffered, suffers) a hypoglycaemic episode. He .... (was failing, had failed, would have failed) to monitor his blood sugar level for more than thirty-six hours and allowed it (dropped, dropping, to drop) to a dangerously low level. Before the episode he .... (would have worked, worked, had been working) physically hard and .... (had been experiencing, were experiencing, to experience) symptoms such as tiredness, irritability and hunger. He .... (did lose, loose, lost) consciousness and fell, though he did not .... (incurred, incurring, incur) injury. He was .... (taken, took, taking) immediately to hospital where treatment .... (gave, given, was given) and he was advised by a nurse about how .... (maintaining, maintained, to maintain) his blood sugar level and .... (avoiding, avoided, to avoid) a repetition of the problem.

Exercise 18h

1 The patient said he had been snapping people's heads off. This means he was:
   a. out of control.
   b. bad tempered.
   c. rude.

2 Before the episode, the patient was:
   a. dressed up.
   b. dressed down.
   c. dressed.

3 When the patient thinks about driving he is:
   a. excited.
   b. alarmed.
   c. amazed.

4 The nurse advised the patient to:
   a. be prepared for an episode.
   b. prepare for an episode.
   c. prepare an episode.

5 The patient forgot to check his blood glucose level because:
   a. he had a lot on.
   b. he didn't have much on.
   c. he had nothing on.

6 Before the nurse left, the patient:
   a. tried to give her something.
   b. tried to sell her something.
   c. tried to buy something from her.

Conversation 18.5: Mourning a friend

This is a conversation in which a woman talks to a nurse about her friend, who has just died. The woman's dialect is that of South Wales.

NURSE: I just want to say how very sorry I am about your friend.

GWYNETH: Ta love.

NURSE: Did it come as a shock?

GWYNETH: No, not really. Getting real bard he was in them last few weeks like. Sinking for months really. Mind you it's been going on frages. In the end he had the gyp chronic. Terrible ramping he was, in his chest like. We wasn't related like, but we was real good friends. Real cut up I am.

NURSE: Yes, it must have been very difficult.

GWYNETH: Well, yes. There was a time twelve-month back when we fancied he was coming better, poor dab. He rallied, you know, for a tidy spell and he was happy then. And we fancied – you know – that he was coming better. Praying for him I was. Of a sudden like he seemed to be bucking up. After there he was full of it and he was coming stronger – little walks around the bailey even and I fancied, 'God is merciful.'

He was under this doctor like, but the doctor warned us not to expect too much – 'remission' he called it. 'Only temporary' he said. I didn't credit him at the time. Didn't want to, I suppose. But he was right. In the end he slipped back. But did he take on? No he never. And of course all of this, it broke my heart. Such a gentleman he was. Generous to a fault. Never a harsh word for anyone.

NURSE: You'll miss him.

GWYNETH: Proper choked I am, I can tell you. Goes right through me it does. Ach a fie! Gone to a better place than this, he has. No swank about him, not a bit of it. Only a simple ashman he was – never made gaffer and no stranger to hard graft but a lovely feeling man. Proper gentleman he was. Give you the shirt off his back if you asked.

He never had no money to play with, always giving it away he was. 'Gwyn', he says to me, 'Gwyn, I'm going to meet my maker and I can't take none of it with me and I want to get my gummel up to meet Him, isn't it?' So in them last few years he sold everything and gave the money away he did. Hardly a stick of furniture left in the place – all sold for those as asked. 'I've had a tidy bit from life', he says. 'I've had me health and strength, two beautiful kids, a loving wife and now I wants to give something back'.

I fancy he learned me a lot, this ashman, I can tell you. A good old stick. More like him and the world would be a better place, isn't it? Isn't that right?

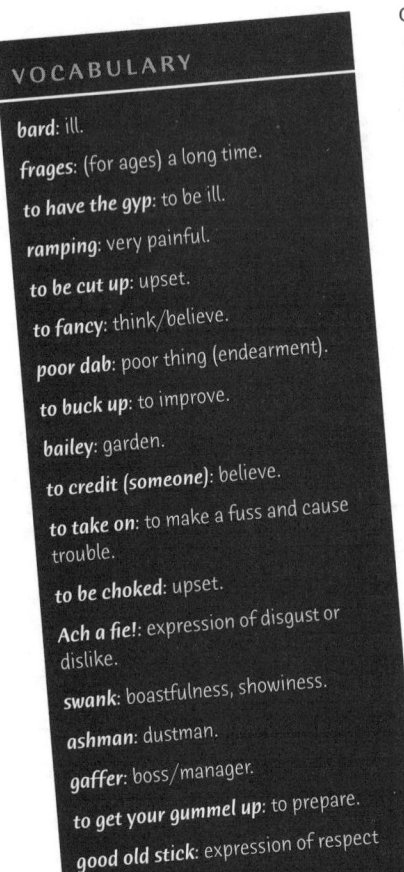

VOCABULARY

bard: ill.

frages: (for ages) a long time.

to have the gyp: to be ill.

ramping: very painful.

to be cut up: upset.

to fancy: think/believe.

poor dab: poor thing (endearment).

to buck up: to improve.

bailey: garden.

to credit (someone): believe.

to take on: to make a fuss and cause trouble.

to be choked: upset.

Ach a fie!: expression of disgust or dislike.

swank: boastfulness, showiness.

ashman: dustman.

gaffer: boss/manager.

to get your gummel up: to prepare.

good old stick: expression of respect and liking.

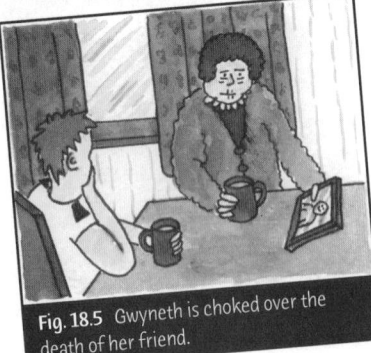

Fig. 18.5 Gwyneth is choked over the death of her friend.

Exercise 18i

From your reading of the conversation, say which of the
following statements are true:

Gwyneth's friend:

a. died suddenly.
b. rallied but relapsed.
c. appeared to get better.
d. didn't accept the doctor's opinion.
e. used to be a manager.
f. refused to become a manager.
g. had no shirt.
h. gave away his furniture.
i. felt sorry for himself.

Exercise 18j

Replace the part of each sentence in brackets with an expression
from a, b or c so that the meaning of the sentence doesn't change:

1 I didn't get up for three days – so (poorly) did I feel.
a. bard
b. gyp
c. cut up

2 All the children were very (distressed) to see their mam in hospital.
a. bucked up
b. full of it
c. choked

3 He just couldn't (accept) the bad news the doctor gave him.
a. credit
b. take up
c. buck up

4 My wife does (nag) so about my cigarette smoking.
a. cut up
b. credit
c. take on

5 I fancy in this hospital there are too many (people in charge) and not
enough workers.
a. ashmen
b. swanks
c. gaffers

6 A (fair time) has passed since the operation and there have been no
complications.
a. frages
b. dead slow period
c. tidy spell

7 He got very little sympathy from his sister who told him to (make an
effort) and stop feeling sorry for himself.
a. buck up
b. take on
c. get his gummel up

Conversation 18.6: A devil of a rash

The following conversation is between a nurse and a patient with possible shingles. The patient uses an Irish dialect.

MR O'NEIL: Will yer look at the rash on me! Here, down the side o' me face. <u>And doesn't it go all the way down me arm too</u>.

NURSE: Let's have a look then. Where is it?

MR O'NEIL [rolling up the sleeve of his shirt]:   It was murder last week but there was no rash then. All I wanted to do was scratch and scratch. Then a couple of days back this rash appears on my arm and then it spreads up here on to the side of my face.

NURSE: Is this the only place? What about the other arm?

MR O'NEIL: No. Just the left side. Look – a straight line. Ah! Careful! It hurts.

NURSE: I see.

MR O'NEIL: And I feel so low. Every day I'm bushed. All day, every day. Well, before the rash appeared I was terrible knackered. Getting run down – me nose full of snot and a cough like a nanny goat. Then this.

NURSE: Have you tried anything for it?

MR O'NEIL: I have, to be sure. But divil could I find a thing of use. Paracetamol? I tried that but it was about as useful as a match on a motorbike. Now there's a bit o' Irish for yer. No, it made no difference at all.

NURSE: This is a nasty one. Here's a blister – up here at the top of your arm.

MR O'NEIL: I know. It hurts, nurse. To tell you the truth, I can't even stand my shirt rubbing against it. What in God's name is it? <u>It's got me flummoxed</u>.

NURSE: Yes. It looks pretty bad. I think you've got shingles. You should see the doctor and I'll make an appointment. Mmm … shingles, certainly looks like it. Mr O'Neil, have you had chickenpox?

MR O'NEIL: When I was a boy, yes. What's shingles?

NURSE: It's a sort of adult chickenpox. Happens when you get run down but you only get it if you've had chickenpox. It starts off as a pain, just as you say you had, then it becomes a rash and then the blisters burst like this one up here. You only get it on one side of your body – just like you've got.

MR O'NEIL: Well, you're a cute one to know all that stuff, to be sure. <u>Will you be after giving me a little something for it?</u>

NURSE: Well, as I say, you'll have to see the doctor first and he'll probably prescribe some kind of painkiller – an anti-inflammatory one. But calamine lotion – you should try calamine lotion – just apply it gently and it might relieve the itching and the soreness.

MR O'NEIL: Well, if it does that it'll be grand. And how long am I going to have this shingles?

NURSE: Oh, I should think you'll be well over it within a week or so. Maybe two weeks.

MR O'NEIL: Would it be catching, this shingles? I mean if it's the chicken pox, that's the <u>divil of a catching thing</u>, isn't it?

NURSE: Shingles is, yes it is. Is there anyone else living in your house?

MR O'NEIL: In the gaff? Me missus, yes and we're with two babbys in the house and all. Will they be getting it then? If herself picks it up she'll <u>eat me head off</u>.

NURSE: It's possible, Mr O'Neil. So it might be best to avoid getting too close for a while until the blisters have dried out in a couple of weeks.

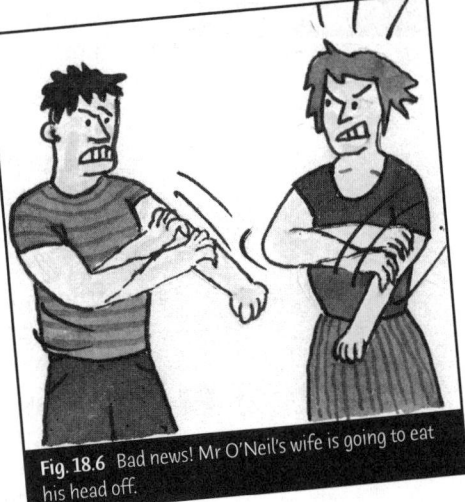

Fig. 18.6 Bad news! Mr O'Neil's wife is going to eat his head off.

MR O'NEIL: Yes, I'm wide to it, so I am. And who would I be catching this shingles from then?

NURSE: Well no one in particular. You can get shingles any time because you've still got the virus in your system from when you were a child and had chickenpox. It happens when people get run down and their immune system isn't working right. You probably need a holiday, Mr O'Neil.

MR O'NEIL: <u>Fat chance!</u> I've got <u>too much on my plate</u> at the moment, so I have.

NURSE: Well you'll have to take some time off.

MR O'NEIL: How long do you reckon?

NURSE: Two weeks, three weeks.

MR O'NEIL: Away on! I can't. I've got bills to pay and mouths to feed, so I have.

Exercise 18k   **Say which of the following statements are true:**

a. Mr O'Neil has a rash only down the side of his face.

b. Mr O'Neil has a rash down only one side of his face.

c. The rash had hurt the previous week.

d. There was no rash a week ago.

e. The rash is two days old.

f. Mr O'Neil feels cheerful.

g. Mr O'Neil feels depressed.

h. Paracetamol has proved useful.

i. The nurse makes a definite diagnosis.

j. Mr O'Neil has had chickenpox.

k. Mr O'Neil has chickenpox.

l. The shingles will be gone after a fortnight.

m. The shingles will be gone in a couple of weeks.

n. According to the nurse, people get shingles after being in an accident.

o. Mr O'Neil is too busy to have a holiday.

p. Mr O'Neil eats too much.

Exercise 18l   **Answer the following questions by choosing an answer from a, b and c:**

1   When Mr O'Neil says, 'and doesn't it go all the way down me arm' he is:
a. asking the nurse to check because he cannot see for himself.
b. pointing the rash out to the nurse.
c. saying that there is no rash.

2   When Mr O'Neil says 'It's got me flummoxed' he means:
a. 'the shingles makes me feel confused.'
b. 'I don't know what the rash is.'
c. 'I don't know anything about shingles.'

3   When asking 'Will you be after giving me a little something for it?' Mr O'Neil wants to know if:
a. the nurse has given him some medicine.
b. any medicine for it exists.
c. he can have some medicine for the shingles.

4   'A divil of a catching thing' is:
a. something very contagious.
b. an unpleasant thing.
c. a dangerous thing.

5   If Mr O'Neil's wife gets chickenpox she will 'eat his head off', in other words she will:
a. devour him.
b. physically attack him.
c. be furious with him.

6   Mr O'Neil has too much on his plate. In other words he:
a. eats too much.
b. is too ill to work.
c. is too busy to stop working.

7   A 'fat chance' is:
a. maybe.
b. a strong possibility.
c. an impossibility.

Conversation 18.7: Belting up

This conversation is between two female patients from Glasgow. They are discussing the problems of living with a colostomy.

ANNE: I'm fair jiggered, I can tell yeh.

MARGARET: Aye, I thought you looked a wee bit <u>peely wally</u>. <u>What's up</u> wi' you?

VOCABULARY

fair: very

jiggered: tired out.

peely wally: pale and sickly.

yon: this.

scunnered: fed up.

get away: you're joking.

letting off: flatulence/wind.

hen: term of endearment like 'love', 'dear' or 'darling'.

to beat about the bush: to go around the subject and not talk direct.

geggy: mouth.

fart: wind.

mind: be careful.

a case: a strange/funny/entertaining person.

(something) and a half: big/a lot.

to have someone on: to fool someone.

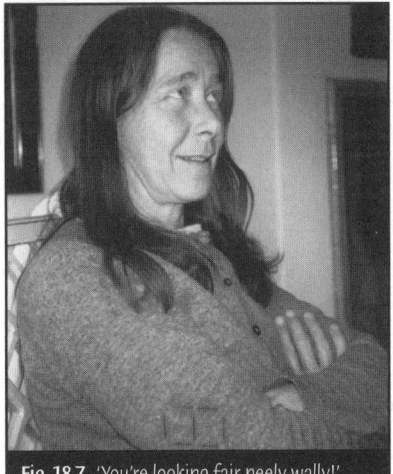

Fig. 18.7 'You're looking fair peely wally!'

ANNE: Och, it's yon colostomy. Fair scunnered with it, so I am.

MARGARET: Why? What's the problem?

ANNE: Well, it's kinda embarrassing. I don't like to talk about it.

MARGARET: Och, gonnae no' be shy with me. See me, see ma bag, had it four years.

ANNE: Get away!

MARGARET: No. It's true. So I know all about it. What's troubling you? Is it <u>letting off?</u> Sorry, hen. What's the word? Wind. Is it wind that's giving you worries? It usually is the worst thing for most folk. There's the noise and the smell.

ANNE: Aye. That's right. You don't <u>beat about the bush</u> do you?

MARGARET: Aye well, my man just tells me to shut ma geggy. But I say life's too short, hen. I <u>cannae be doing</u> with what people are going to think.

ANNE: Aye, well. Have you got any advice then? What can I do about it?

MARGARET: Food. Watch what you eat – that's the first thing – the doctor has probably told you that – but even then the wind is difficult to control. But ma mam had a good idea about the farting noise. She has went and bought a nurse's belt. Know what I mean? One o' they elasticated belts?

ANNE: Aye?

MARGARET: She got it from one of they <u>wee</u> charity shops in Dumbarton Road. Saw it in the window, bought it for me. If you wear it round your waist, under your clothes and put it so it covers the bag – not too tight <u>mind</u>, just enough – and it keeps down the noise. You won't hear a thing, honest. Quiet as a whisper, your farts will be.

ANNE [LAUGHING]:   You are a case <u>and a half</u>. You're not <u>having me on?</u>

MARGARET [LAUGHING]:   Never! Trust me. Try it for yourself and see.

Exercise 18m

Choose a word from a, b and c to replace the word or phrase in brackets in the following sentences:

1   What's (up)?
a. the matter
b. on
c. out

2   She looks (fair peely wally).
a. pretty bad.
b. a little off colour.
c. tip top.

3   The patient is embarrassed about (letting off.)
a. smelling.
b. smells herself.
c. smelly.

4   She (cannae be doing) with other people's opinions.
a. doesn't care
b. can't be bothered
c. isn't worried

5   The doctor prescribed a (wee bit) of medicine.
a. small
b. little
c. small amount

6   Waiting (isn't half) boring.
a. isn't a bit
b. is very
c. is not really

7   I thought the doctor was (having me on) when he said I could go home.
a. lying
b. cheating
c. laughing

8   (Mind) you don't tie it too tightly.
a. Care
b. Carefully
c. Watch

9   The problem is (kinda) difficult to describe.
a. sort of
b. not
c. little

10   Tell me the facts and don't (beat around the bush).
a. tell me directly.
b. avoid the truth.
c. tell me the truth.

Answers and Comments on the Language.

Exercise 18a

b.

e.

f. 'mucking about' usually means 'messing around/clowning/not being serious'. It can also mean (as it means here) 'to try, in a light-hearted way, to make someone believe something that is not true'.

Exercise 18b

1   b. Mr Parker's answer 'No' is in response to the nurse's question 'I hope you don't mind…' So his answer means 'No I don't mind.' In other words, 'yes'.

2   b.

3   b.

4   a.

5   b.

6   c.

7   b.

8   c.

9   a.

Exercise 18c

1   a.

2   b.

3   c.

4   c.

5   b.

6   c.

7   a.

Exercise 18d

1   c.

2   a.

3   c.

4   a.

5   a.

6   a.

7   c.

Exercise 18e

1   **c.** 'It's time' means 'now is the right moment.'

2   **a.** 'Over-staffed' (option **c**) means there are too many people working. It is the opposite of 'under-staffed'.

3   **b.** 'Chores' are everyday routine jobs. You can 'give' a hand or 'lend' a hand to mean 'help'.

4   **b.** To 'cop' can mean to 'look at'. 'Cop a load of this' means 'look at this'.

5   **c.** In non-standard English, often verbs are used which look like the present tense but which are, in fact, telling something about the past.

6   **c.**

7   **c.** 'To end up' is often used when talking about a bad future or destiny. For example, 'You will end up in hospital if you keep drinking like that.'

8   **c.**

Exercise 18f

The following statements are true:

b. The word 'smelly' almost always refers to a *bad* smell.

e.

f.

g.

i.

j.

Exercise 18g

Mr John Clarke <u>suffered</u> a hypoglycaemic episode. He <u>had failed</u> to monitor his blood sugar level for more than thirty-six hours and allowed it <u>to drop</u> to a dangerously low level. Before the episode, he <u>had been working</u> physically hard and <u>had been experiencing</u> symptoms such as tiredness, irritability and hunger. He <u>lost</u> consciousness and fell though he did not <u>incur</u> injury. He was <u>taken</u> immediately to hospital where treatment <u>was given</u> and he was advised by a nurse about how <u>to maintain</u> his blood sugar level and <u>to avoid</u> a repetition of the problem.

Exercise 18h

1   **b.**

2   **a.** 'To be dressed up' is to be wearing smart clothes.

3   **b.** 'To be alarmed' is to be very worried. Hospitals commonly issue statements about patients such as 'there is no cause for alarm'.

4   a. This sentence suggests that the patient doesn't know if or when an episode will occur.

5   a. 'To have something on' means to be involved in something/to be busy.

6   b.

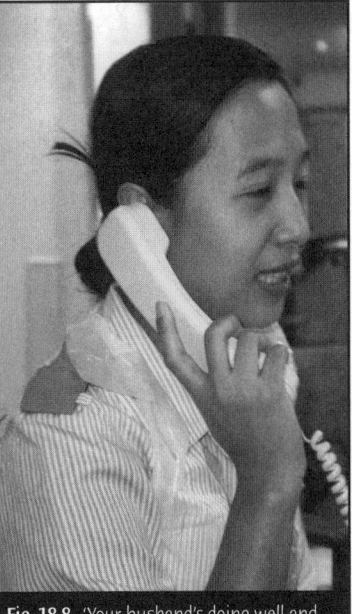

Fig. 18.8 'Your husband's doing well and there's no cause for alarm.'

Exercise 18i

Both **b** and **c** are true.

'To rally' (statement **b**) means 'to become stronger'.

It is Gwyneth who does not accept the doctor's prognosis (statement **d**), not her friend.

Her friend 'never made gaffer' (did not become a manager) but there is nothing in what she says to suggest he refused to become one (statement **f**).

The expression 'to give the shirt off (your) back' refers to generosity, but is only an expression and not a literal truth (statement **g**). 'To lose the shirt off (your) back' means 'to lose everything'.

Gwyneth's friend sold his furniture, he did not 'give it away' for free (statement **h**).

Gwyneth says her friend didn't 'take on'. In other words he didn't complain or feel sorry for himself (statement **i**).

Exercise 18j

1   a.
2   c.
3   a.
4   c.
5   c.
6   c.
7   a.

Exercise 18k

The following statements are true:

b. The important thing to note is the position of the word 'only' in both statements **a** and **b**.

d.

e. 'A couple of days back' means 'two days ago'.

g. Mr O'Neil describes his symptoms as feeling low (depressed) and knackered (tired).

j. 'Has had chickenpox' means he had it once in the past but no longer has it.

l.

m.

o.

Exercise 18l

1   b.

2   b.

3   c.

4   a.

5   c.

6   c.

7   c.

Exercise 18m

1   a. 'What's on?' (option **b**) means 'What's happening?'

2   a.

3   a.

4   b. Note that 'can't be bothered' (option **b**) is followed by 'about' or 'with' or 'by'.

5   c.

6   c.

7   a.

8   c.

9   a.

10   b.